# Sickness, Stigma and ...wakening

# Sickness, Stigma and Spiritual Awakening

A Transpersonal Paradigm for Women with Contested Illnesses

**Bernadette Masterson**

PETER LANG

Oxford • Bern • Berlin • Bruxelles • New York • Wien

Bibliographic information published by Die Deutsche Bibliothek
Die Deutsche Bibliothek lists this publication in the Deutsche Nationalbibliografie;
detailed bibliographic data is available on the Internet at http://dnb.ddb.de.

A catalogue record for this book is available at the British Library.

Library of Congress Cataloging-in-Publication Data: A CIP catalog record for this book
has been applied for at the Library of Congress.

Cover image: Woman in tall ferns by A L L E F . V I N I C I U S Δ on Unsplash. Free for
commercial use.

ISBN 978-1-78874-341-9 (print) • ISBN 978-1-78874-342-6 (ePDF)
ISBN 978-1-78874-343-3 (ePub) • ISBN 978-1-78874-344-0 (mobi)

© Peter Lang AG 2019

Published by Peter Lang Ltd, International Academic Publishers,
52 St Giles, Oxford, OX1 3LU, United Kingdom
oxford@peterlang.com, www.peterlang.com

Bernadette Masterson has asserted her right under the Copyright, Designs and Patents
Act, 1988, to be identified as Author of this Work.

Printed in Germany

# Contents

# Preface

When a person who has enjoyed good health becomes ill, they are likely to experience a range of emotional responses: anxiety about their diagnosis, lack of knowledge around potential medical interventions, uncertainty in relation to their on-going care and management of their condition and the possible consequences for their lifestyle and their family. These experiences are heightened if their interaction with the health system and healthcare professionals is not positive. And, it is especially difficult when a person suffers from an illness that is contested – where their symptoms and diagnosis are challenged by health professionals – and their lived experience is not believed. However, as this book attests, the cloud of anguish and suffering that arises from such contestation can also have a silver lining – it can give rise to an experience of spiritual awakening in the one who suffers.

In this ground-breaking work, Bernadette Masterson explores the nature of the phenomenon of spiritual awakening amongst women, with physical illnesses which are invisible and chronic and who have been subject to disbelief by healthcare professionals, family and friends. This very timely book brings together and examines an extensive body of research on the topic in light of the experience of nine women with chronic invisible illness. The book is especially powerful because it gives a deep and rich account of the experiences and suffering of these women and assesses the traumatic impact on their lives, relationships and well-being of not being believed.

While this work will be of interest to the general reader and, in particular, those who experience a contested illness, it has special relevance for healthcare professionals; it presents a particular challenge to those engaged in the training of healthcare professionals. It highlights the need for the development in the medical humanities of a model which is respectful of the experience of invisible illnesses and which acknowledges the potential of such experiences for spiritual awakening.

This book provides compelling evidence for a narrative approach to medical practice and stresses the importance of attentive listening and narrative competence as key elements in medical training. Such advice is supported by the Guide to Professional Conduct and Ethics of the Irish Medical Council[1] which reminds us that doctors must always be guided by their primary responsibility to act in the best interests of their patients. Such a narrative approach is also congruent with the definition of professionalism of the Royal College of Surgeons in Ireland which acknowledges the need for a partnership between patient and doctor which is based, inter alia, on reflective practice leading to greater self-awareness in the medical practitioner and grounded in mutual respect.[2] This book should prove to be particularly valuable to the medical profession as a means of fashioning more compassionate clinical engagement with patients and as an aid to generate amongst its members an appreciation of the benefits of phenomenology and of narrative medicine as supplementary diagnostic tools.

The chapters on spiritual awakening in this book are particularly illuminating. Bernadette's exploration of spiritual awakening in light of historical and contemporary spiritual writers and the interdisciplinary field of the medical humanities is particularly useful. Pellegrino, one of the founding fathers of the medical humanities, argued that the *wounded humanity* of patients must be seen and understood by the medical profession. This wounding occurs because patients suffer from the loss of three basic freedoms – freedom of action, freedom to make rational choices and freedom from the power of others – and the loss of a sense of the integrity of the self. Bernadette's research suggests, however, that women may be empowered by considering illness as a possible gateway to spiritual awakening, as a call to a more contemplative, wisdom way of being. As she expresses it herself: 'The idea of illness as a contemplative path offers a hopeful paradigm ... leading individuals from oppression and illness to liberation and healing.'

Bernadette explores how Assagioli's theory of psychosynthesis, the writings of women mystics and scholars from the field of medical humanities

---

1    *Guide to Professional Conduct and Ethics for Registered Medical Practitioners* (8th Edition, 2016).
2    *Medical Professionalism: Promoting Patient and Physician Safety* (RCSI, 2018). See also: *Transforming Healthcare Education, Research and Service: RCSI Strategic Plan 2018–2022.*

can illuminate the mechanism of inner awakening experienced by the participants in her research. She develops an innovative, heuristic, seven-stage model of the journey of such spiritual awakening which is grounded in the themes emerging from her research. The model represents milestones on the women's journey through the landscape of chronic invisible illness toward a mystical inner awakening and a wisdom way of being.

This book also offers support to carers, family and friends – as well as therapists and spiritual directors – by helping them to gain a deeper understanding of the extent of shame, stigma and trauma experienced by sufferers of chronic contested illnesses. Such understanding can lead to more compassionate support for the suffering patient.

In recent decades there has been a growing awareness within the healthcare professions about the importance of spiritual care. This intelligent, well-researched and very readable book makes an important and timely contribution to that ongoing dialogue.

David Smith
Associate Professor of Healthcare Ethics
Royal College of Surgeons in Ireland

# Illustrations

# Acknowledgements

This book has been a long time in the making, and could not have been accomplished without the encouragement, guidance and inspiration of a number of people. Firstly, I want to thank the women who took part in the original research with such generosity of spirit. In the face of ill health, they were willing to sacrifice scarce energy resources in order to convey with courage, humility and honesty, their inner worlds of meaning-making whilst living with chronic contested illnesses. For reasons of confidentiality, I am not in a position to thank them by name. My sole offering in return is dedicating this book to them.

I am indebted to Bernadette Flanagan whose support for this topic has been unwavering since our first meeting. Without her commitment at that time as head of research at All Hallows College, Dublin City University, the project would not have come to pass. I was truly privileged to have had Bernadette, an international pioneer in the academic study of spirituality, as both mentor and supervisor for the doctoral study. I have had the good fortune also to have the co-operation and encouragement of Michael O'Sullivan not only in the formative years of this endeavour, but also more recently as colleague and director of the Spirituality Institute for Research and Education (SpIRE).

Noel Keating has supported me with great patience and skill in the process of writing the book and I am most grateful to him for his time, his insights, and his wise observations.

My thanks to Christabel Scaife who was my first point of contact at Peter Lang. Her hospitality towards the book proposal was heartening. Anthony Mason, also of Peter Lang, has been affirming from the start, and gracious in his responses to the diverse queries foisted upon him. Working with Peter Lang has been, all along, a positive and uplifting experience.

A very special thanks to my friend Anne Hederman, without whom this book would not have seen the light of day. Crucial also was support and encouragement from Raymond Cadwell, Michele Ryan, João Sita,

Gabrielle Jin, Karen Ward, Orla McMahon, Camilla Powell, and Helene Vania. Gratitude is owed to Steven Singleton for his kindness and unwavering patience in assisting with electronic referencing; sincere thanks also to Éibhlís Nic Uaithuas for skilful input with word processing matters.

Finally, in terms of practical care and support from family, I thank my sister, Maura, for hearty meals, and my brother, Brian, for biomagnetic therapy treatments, all of which contributed to generating vital energy for the completion of the book.

# Introduction

This book is based on a PhD study which employed a narrative framework to research the nature of the phenomenon of spiritual awakening amongst ten women (including the author) who experience chronic 'invisible' physical illnesses. The term *invisible illness* applies to illnesses which are, or have been, contested in relation to their validity as genuine physical conditions. These disorders have been a subject of dispute in medical practice and, consequently, amongst elements of the media and in society. Standard laboratory testing returns a negative result, rendering them 'invisible' in a medical context. Invisibility is reinforced when the bearers of such conditions may appear to look well on the occasions when they appear in public. The principal types of invisible or contested illnesses featured in this research include:

1. Myalgic Encephalomyelitis (ME) which is also called Chronic Fatigue Syndrome (CFS), Post-Viral Syndrome, and Systematic Exertion Intolerance Disease (SEID)
2. Fibromyalgia
3. Chronic Lyme Disease
4. Multiple Chemical Sensitivity
5. Electro-Sensitivity

Positioned in the field of medical humanities, this study introduces into the field the possibility of affirming a life-giving spiritual paradigm for the journey through chronic invisible illnesses by exploring, through a psycho-spiritual lens, the illness narratives of ten women.

## Personal Context for the Research

A brief outline here of my own experience of spiritual awakening in chronic invisible illness may illuminate my decision to research this topic. The key components embedded in the title of this book have been an intrinsic part of my personal narrative. Indeed, my own ongoing fluctuating health challenges have informed this reflexive study and are woven into its fabric, enfolding the concept of illness as a bearer of wisdom.

Firstly, I developed an interest in the topic of spiritual awakening in chronic invisible illness as a result of having life-long challenges with it. As a child, I had a congenital heart defect, a large Patent Ductus Arteriosus (PDA). This wasn't discovered until I was five. A large PDA that remains open for an extended time can cause the heart to enlarge, forcing it to work harder. Also, fluid can build up in the lungs.[1] The family doctor misdiagnosed the sounds emanating from my lungs as chest infections. My mother recalled in later years that I had been on antibiotics 'non-stop' up until the age of five. The school doctor discovered the PDA and in 1964 I was sent for heart surgery for a PDA and enlarged heart which at the time entailed an eight-week traumatising hospital stay. After that, my heart was thankfully in order but I was euphemistically labelled 'delicate', being prone to bouts of illness and exhaustion all of my life. For many years in adult life, without satisfactory diagnosis or treatment and trying to sustain a demanding career in London, I frequented a range of complementary medicine practitioners. From my first association with complementary healing, I underwent a transformation of my worldview as a result of the treatments themselves, and subsequent personal research on the paradigmatic underpinnings of each chosen healing modality. This journey was my initial spiritual awakening in chronic invisible illness.

Secondly, I was motivated by personal experiences during a six-year period when my health had deteriorated to the extent that I could not work,

---

1    PubMed Health, 'Patent Ductus Arteriosus', *PubMed Health*, 11 June 2014, <https://www.ncbi.nlm.nih.gov/pubmedhealth/PMH0062968/>.

feeling alone and isolated with a chronic invisible illness. My chief support system then presented itself in an informal, mainly telephone-based, support group of women with conditions similar to mine. Like me, these women felt marginalised and stigmatised because of contestation, amongst some elements of the medical profession and the popular media, that the nature of the illness was not physical but psychological in aetiology. More shaming still were associations of their types of illnesses with malingering.

Yet the compassion, the attentive presence, the wisdom, the grace, and the generosity in the face of chronic ill-health demonstrated by these women have left a lasting impression on me. In addition, a numinous ambience often infused the atmosphere during my interactions with this cohort of women. Having trained in psychosynthesis, a psycho-spiritual psychology, a curiosity blossomed within my mind concerning the nature of this quality of presence which I considered might point to a spiritual awakening that had occurred on their illness journey.

I was reminded by this presence of occasions when Roger Evans, my wise and gifted teacher at the Institute of Psychosynthesis in London, endeavoured to describe a sublime spiritual quality which presented itself, for example, in a group setting, or when he was trying to convey a sense of deep wonder or sacred mystery that proved ineffable to the most eloquent. Resorting to a hand gesture, Roger used to extend his hand and delicately stroke his thumb against his forefinger and middle finger, as though he were momentarily caressing some kind of precious diamond dust to convey its exquisiteness. With this heuristic gesticulation Roger would ask us, 'Do you get a sense of that? Do you get a feel for that?' Like Roger, I tried to get a sense of, a feel for, the phenomenon of this quality, this exquisite numinous energy that permeated encounters with these women who had supported me.

Pilgrimage journeys to India, Brazil and Medjugorje in pursuit of healing led to encounters with other travellers with chronic invisible, contested illnesses who, also in search of that elusive cure and deeper peace, demonstrated similar qualities. It appeared to me that they had reached a level of consciousness that afforded little or no judgement, was inclusive, wise, and beyond the ordinary.

These incidents inspired me to explore and convey 'a sense of that, a feel for that' – that phenomenon of spiritual awakening in chronic invisible illnesses. I was also inspired to reflect on the potential of such an exploration for redressing the perception of the dominant discourses of medicine in which illness is perceived as purely a negative circumstance. A more hopeful paradigm of illness, for those who experience it, might be enabled to flourish if difficult illness experiences could be reframed as potential bearers of wisdom as well as gateways to spiritual awakening.

This study set out with the single aim of exploring 'what is the nature of the phenomenon of spiritual awakening amongst women, with physical illnesses which are invisible and chronic, and who have been subjected to disbelief?' Its intention was to find out more about the features of awakening and the connection between illness, isolation, disbelief and the occurrence of the awakening itself.

## The Nature of the Study

The study is founded on post-positivist principles which assert that all observation is biased and which reject the idea that a person can see the world as it really is. The heuristic exploratory methodological approach employed here is underpinned by transpersonal theory and research methods, and acknowledges the self of the researcher as the chief instrument of inquiry. Central to the study was the creation of the researcher's own narrative of illness, its analysis, and the application of its findings in the analysis of illness narratives of nine other women. This approach is in keeping with Romanyshyn's notion of the 'wounded researcher', holding that personal psychological exploration is a pre-requisite for in-depth psychological research on others.[2] The exploratory strategy encompassed a blend of qualitative methods including narrative inquiry, intuitive inquiry, reflexivity, phenomenology, psycho-spiritual psychology, and hermeneutics.

2    R. Romanyshyn, *The Wounded Researcher: Research with Soul in Mind* (New Orleans, LA: Spring Journal, Inc., 2007), 209.

This work lies within a feminist paradigm in so far as its methodology has been influenced by intuitive inquiry, the transpersonal research method developed by Rosemarie Anderson, which in turn was influenced in its development by feminist theory and research practices.[3] Intuitive inquiry is an epistemology of the heart that seeks to combine intuition with intellectual precision. It seeks transformation in the researcher and participants alike. The work lies within the framework of Standpoint Feminism, a theory which emerged in the 1970s, influenced by Marxism, challenging androcentric, economically advantaged, racist, and Eurocentric conceptual frameworks.[4] Standpoint Feminist theory holds that marginalised groups of women with distinct experiences are socially situated in ways that make it more possible for them to be aware of their specific experiences, and to ask questions about them, than it is for the non-marginalised. This research also falls within the domain of feminist spirituality as espoused by Constance Fitzgerald and Beverly Lanzetta, both of whom share the outlook of Teresa of Avila as a 'cartographer of the soul' who explored the contemplative process that brought her, as a marginalised female, from fragmentation to a sense of dignity in a male-dominated Church.[5]

## Contribution to the Literature

Although there has been a burgeoning in the literature on spirituality and health,[6] this research endeavour was unable to locate any research encompassing a psycho-spiritual exploration of spiritual awakening or spiritual

---

3   R. Anderson, 'Intuitive Inquiry: An Epistemology of the Heart for Scientific Inquiry', *The Humanistic Psychologist* 32, no. 4 (2004): 307–41.

4   S. Harding, ed., *The Feminist Standpoint Theory Reader: Intellectual and Political Controversies*, 1st edn (New York: Routledge, 2003), 5.

5   B. Lanzetta, *Radical Wisdom: A Feminist Mystical Theology* (Minneapolis, MN: Fortress Press, 2005), 99.

6   Harold Koenig of Duke University, North Carolina, has published a comprehensive overview of the research on religion, spirituality and health. See: H. Koenig,

development in chronic invisible illnesses or indeed in any chronic illness. One study produced by Justin Chernow entitled 'The blessing of a curse: an examination of growth and transformation from chronic fatigue syndrome',[7] which emerged from the transpersonal university Sophia in Palo Alto, California, in 2008, addressed the transformative function of adversity in chronic fatigue syndrome; however, theories of spiritual awakening were not employed as a lens to examine growth and transformation.

An expansion in narratives of illness has been acknowledged by Arthur Frank, professor emeritus of sociology at the University of Calgary, who penned *The Wounded Storyteller* in 1997.[8] Many of the popular narratives of illness pertain to how the authors gained wisdom, insights and spiritual awakening in illness. A journal article entitled 'Sacred illness: exploring transpersonal aspects in physical affliction and the role of the body in spiritual development', by Ellis Linders and Les Lancaster of Liverpool John Moores University, was published in the British journal *Mental Health, Religion and Culture* in 2013. In this article, the authors commented on the difficulty in locating literature on the topic of spiritual development and the body: 'Whilst the occurrence of psychological upheaval accompanying spiritual development is given much attention in the relevant literature, physical involvement in transpersonal experience is a relatively uncharted area.'[9]

Mary Vachon has argued that cancer can lead to a spiritual awakening which can be seen as a form of alchemy. Her paper provides qualitative descriptions of the 'field' or 'soul wisdom' experienced by patients and

---

*Handbook of Religion and Health* (Oxford; New York: Oxford University Press, 2012).

7    J. Chernow, 'The Blessing of a Curse: An Examination of Growth and Transformation from Chronic Fatigue Syndrome' (Institute of Transpersonal Psychology, 2008), <http://gradworks.umi.com/33/07/3307970.html>.

8    A. Frank, *The Wounded Storyteller: Body, Illness, and Ethics*, pbk edn (Chicago: University of Chicago Press, 1997).

9    L. Lancaster and E. Linders, 'Sacred Illness: Exploring Transpersonal Aspects in Physical Affliction and the Role of the Body in Spiritual Development', *Mental Health* 16, no. 10 (2013): 991–1008, <https://doi.org/10.1080/13674676.2012.728578>.

caregivers.[10] While there is an interesting body of narrative qualitative research in the field of women and chronic illness,[11] none of it refers to the possible 'spiritual awakening' gateway which may be accessed in chronic illness; though themes associated with use of already available spiritual resources are engaged. *Embodiment and the Search for Illness Legitimacy among Women* is the title of a 2005 study of eighteen women in Michigan which examined how narratives provide a window on the way in which women with contested illnesses negotiated a sense of human value and belonging.[12] The stories these women told highlight medicine's limitations in describing the contested illness experience and illustrate how important it was for them to make sense of illness in relation to, and with, others, especially with other individuals with contested illnesses. A further study on chronic ill health in 2009 from Norway called *Narrative-In-Action in Women with Chronic Rheumatic Conditions* used a hermeneutic approach to study meaning-making processes in the narratives of six women, and has a focus on how society's labelling mechanisms impact upon the women's everyday lives.[13]

The themes of chronic illness, spirituality and healing have been brought together in a collection of essays edited by Stoltzfus et al. in interdisciplinary,

10    M. Vachon, 'The Soul's Wisdom: Stories of Living and Dying', *Current Oncology* 15, no. 0 (2008): 48–52, <https://doi.org/10.3747/co.v15i0.272>.

11    A. Werner, L. Widding Isaksen, and K. Malterud, '"I Am Not the Kind of Woman Who Complains of Everything": Illness Stories on Self and Shame in Women with Chronic Pain', *Social Science & Medicine* 59 (2004): 1035–45; D. Kralik, 'The Quest for Ordinariness: Transition Experienced by Midlife Women Living with Chronic Illness', *Journal of Advanced Nursing* 39, no. 2 (1 July 2002): 146–54, doi:10.1046/j.1365-2648.2000.02254.x; B. Rasmussen et al., 'Young Women With Type 1 Diabetes' Management of Turning Points and Transitions', *Qualitative Health Research* 17, no. 3 (1 March 2007): 300–10, doi:10.1177/1049732306298631.

12    D. Swoboda, 'Embodiment and the Search for Illness Legitimacy Among Women with Contested Illnesses', *Michigan Feminist Studies* 19 (Fall 2005): 73–90.

13    S. Alsaker, *Narrative in Action: Meaning-Making in Everyday Activities of Women Living with Chronic Rheumatic Conditions* (Norges teknisk-naturvitenskapelige universitet, Fakultet for samfunnsvitenskap og teknologiledelse, Institutt for sosialt arbeid og helsevitenskap, 2009), <http://brage.bibsys.no/xmlui/handle/11250/267660>.

religious and intercultural perspectives.[14] Stoltzfus, Professor of Religion at Georgia Gwinnett College since 2015, has a particular research interest in examining how diverse religions represent and respond to chronic illness, and what ideas and resources individuals may have in their spiritual traditions that will be of support in chronic illness. The editors' expressed intention is to 'foster inter-religious, cross-cultural, and trans-disciplinary dialogue about chronic illness, spirituality, and healing and to cultivate creative ways to respond and relate to the fragile yet resilient human condition.'[15]

One of the contributions consists of a narrative of her own illness experience by Ruth Krall, Emeritus Professor of Religion, Psychology and Nursing at Goshen College, Indiana. Krall was diagnosed as having endometrial cancer in 1995. Her chapter describes her initial shock at her own condemnation of her body and her search for a sense of herself as a whole person. She describes how she found support in the myth of the Sumerian Goddess Inanna whose journey into the underworld of suffering and death was her initiation to a deeper level of consciousness. Much interesting narrative qualitative research has been conducted on women's spirituality.[16] A study of six women, aged eighty and over, carried out by Lydia Manning, gerontologist at Concordia University in Chicago, focused on the spirituality of women in advanced years. This study, which is titled *Spirituality as a Lived Experience: Exploring the Essence of Spirituality for Women in Late Life* provides insights into the nature of the women's lived experiences of

---

14    M. Stoltzfus, R. Green, and D. Schumm, eds, *Chronic Illness, Spirituality, and Healing: Diverse Disciplinary, Religious, and Cultural Perspectives*, 1st edn (New York: Palgrave Macmillan, 2013).

15    Ibid., 11.

16    See D. Schneider, 'The Miracle Bearers: Narratives of Birthing Women and Implications for Spiritually Informed Social Work Practice,' *Journal of Social Service Research* 38, no. 2 (1 January 2012): 212–30, doi:10.1080/01488376.2011.647983; L. Callister and I. Khalaf, 'Spirituality in Childbearing Women,' *The Journal of Perinatal Education* 19, no. 2 (2010): 16–24, doi:10.1624/105812410X495514; J. Mattis, 'African American Women's Definitions of Spirituality and Religiosity,' *Journal of Black Psychology* 26, no. 1 (1 February 2000): 101–22, doi:10.1177/0095798400026001006; F. Wambura Ngunjiri, *Women's Spiritual Leadership in Africa: Tempered Radicals and Critical Servant Leaders* (Albany: State University of New York Press, 2010).

spirituality.[17] It is uncommon, however, to locate a study which attends in a specific manner to the spiritual awakening phase in the spiritual development of women. One exception is a qualitative narrative study titled *A Narrative Inquiry of Women Practitioners of Eastern Spirituality in Recovery from Childhood Trauma*, conducted by Eva Zimmermann at the California Institute of Integral Studies (2011).[18] This examined the experiences of ten women childhood trauma survivors in relation to their psychological growth and pays significant attention to the spiritual awakening component. The trauma emphasised here stemmed from childhood experiences, and spiritual awakening occurred by means of psychotherapeutic methods as well as meditation practices.

The present study, therefore, adds to the literature, and aims to act as a catalyst for further research, by exploring spiritual awakening amongst women with chronic invisible illnesses employing lenses which include the psychosynthesis model developed by Roberto Assagioli together with the work of some other key theorists who have investigated the nature of the spiritual journey of women throughout time. These scholars include Evelyn Underhill, Beverly Lanzetta, Teresa of Avila, Maria Harris, Maureen Murdock, and Bernadette Flanagan.

## Scope

This study has been bounded geographically within the perimeters of the Republic of Ireland. Convenience and snowballing sampling techniques influenced the selection of nine participants whose ages ranged in age from

---

17    L. Manning, 'Spirituality as a Lived Experience: Exploring the Essence of Spirituality for Women in Late Life', *International Journal of Aging & Human Development* 75, no. 2 (2012): 95–113.

18    E. Zimmermann, 'A Narrative Inquiry of Women Practitioners of Eastern Spirituality in Recovery from Childhood Trauma' (California Institute of Integral Studies, 2011), <http://gradworks.umi.com/34/90/3490158.html>. Accessed 28 January 2016.

fifty-two to seventy-one years. While inclusion criteria did not feature educational standards, participants had all completed education to minimum of second level. Interviews were conducted in 2013, the year Ireland ranked fourteenth place in the Euro Health Consumer Index.[19] The time period covering the illness experiences of the participants spanned from 1959 to 2013.

One of the selection criteria for participants in this study was the possession of an interest in spirituality. The researcher acknowledges that all invisible illness may not be accompanied by spiritual awakening. However, it is beyond the boundaries of this study to explore non-awakening as a feature of the illness experience.

This endeavour is not about the experiences of women mystics who were ill, although the narratives of some of the Christian mystics are drawn upon. Although the study concerns *spiritual* awakening, the reader should bear in mind that the theoretical frameworks underpinning the study are not derived from theology – but instead are informed by psycho-spiritual theory as presented in selected interdisciplinary literature. This choice is in line with the characteristic interdisciplinary nature of the academic study of spirituality whereby an investigation may be grounded in a selection of diverse disciplines including literature, psychology, the arts, social science, biology or other disciplines, including theology.

It is beyond the scope of this study to engage in depth with prevailing controversies concerning whether or not invisible illnesses/contested illnesses are physical or psychological in aetiology. In the spirit of narrative inquiry, this research acknowledges the validity of the stories people tell of their illnesses and the window such narratives offer to our culture; sociologist Arthur Frank has argued that telling one's story of illness is a way of re-drawing old maps and finding new destinations and that, 'stories have to *repair* the damage that illness has done to the ill person's sense of where she is in life, and where she may be going.'[20]

---

19    <http://www.irishtimes.com/news/health/irish-emergency-care-waiting-times-rated-worst-in-europe-1.2510236>.

20    Frank, *The Wounded Storyteller*, 53.

For an introduction to the territory of invisible, contested illnesses, the reader is referred to the work of Christine Dancey and Megan Arroll, participants in the University of East London's chronic illness research team, who have analysed the controversies, theories and research surrounding such long-term conditions.[21]

Whilst engaged in the doctoral research, I discovered impressive literature in the self-help/illness narrative genre penned by women with invisible illnesses, writing which was deeply authentic, forthright, and devoid of pretence. In particular Kat Duff's *The Alchemy of Illness* encouraged me along as a perspective on healing which resonated with my own.[22] Having spent two years in bed with CFIDS, this psychotherapist's legacy of her illness is a gem of a collection of candid, reflective essays exploring the notion that every illness is a crucible that tests us, transforms us, and provides us with unique lessons to integrate into our everyday lives. Like Kat, the women I interviewed spoke with courage, inspirational frankness and clarity about their experiences and their insights. Their voices carry a wisdom that is lacking in the world of 'nine-to-five' and offer a sense of meaning and solidarity for others who are ill and disbelieved.

The next chapter, Chapter 1, traces the historical roots of medical humanities, the interdisciplinary field in which this inquiry is positioned. The raison d'être of medical humanities helps to illuminate experiences of women with contested illnesses who speak of feeling invalidated and dismissed. Chapter 2 focuses on two internationally renowned medical doctors – scholars who have set about addressing a perceived lack of empathy in certain areas of medical practice; they advocate a narrative approach in medicine, calling for narrative competence amongst doctors and emphasising the positive impact of doctors' attentive listening to the patient's experience of illness. Chapter 3 assesses the traumatic impact of having a chronic invisible/contested illness, distilling the nature of the trauma peculiar to the kinds of contested illness experiences which featured in the research. Here, the nine women are introduced, and they themselves speak of their

---

21    M. Arroll and C. Dancey, *Invisible Illness: Coping with Misunderstood Conditions* (London: Sheldon Press, 2014).

22    K. Duff, *The Alchemy of Illness* (New York: Harmony, 2000).

experiences of not being believed by doctors recounting the knock-on consequences of this disbelief on their wellbeing and relationships. Chapter 4 presents my foundational theorists on the topic of spiritual awakening. In Chapter 5, the features of spiritual awakening which occurred in the lives of the women are described. Chapter 6 offers an overview of key themes emerging from the research project as a whole. A heuristic model of spiritual awakening for women with chronic invisible experiences is offered in Chapter 7. Some final reflections on the study, its implications and possible applications are considered in Chapter 8. Finally, an outline of the methodological approach utilised is given in the Appendix.

This book seeks to give a voice to a marginalised group of wise women to whom I am indebted; they still have the illnesses while I straddle the worlds of the sick and the well. It is hoped that this exploratory study has the potential to serve as a catalysing force in the evolution of a paradigm in medicine which acknowledges invisible illness as a bearer of possibilities for spiritual awakening, a paradigm which is respectful of invisible illness experiences and which is also life-giving for those who have those illness experiences. It is the central task of medical humanities to humanise medical practice.

# CHAPTER I

# Historical Context: Science at the Expense of Empathy

> I had big relationship problems in my family because some people didn't believe me. Because when the doctors couldn't find anything, some people in my family said, 'Well if the doctors can't find anything there mustn't be anything there, so it must be psychological.' And then all your support is kind of falling away.
>
> — ORLA

The history of medical humanities and the reasons for forming this academic field help to illuminate how it has come to pass that individuals with certain types of debilitating illnesses find that they are not believed by their doctors – disbelief which may have devastating and traumatising knock-on consequences, personal and financial. Accordingly, the interdisciplinary field of medical humanities has been selected as the appropriate arena for the exploration of spiritual awakening in chronic invisible illness. Indeed, medical humanities came into being in the 1970s in response to an over-emphasis on scientific method in medicine, which relegated human contact, and empathy with the suffering patient, to an inferior position. This evolving field which aims to bridge the long-standing gap between medicine and the humanities initially adopted a purpose of facilitating doctors in the understanding of human suffering. Its founding father, Edmund Pellegrino (1920–2013), one of the founders of bioethics, served as president of the Catholic University of America and subsequently as Professor of Medicine and Medical Ethics at the Georgetown Medical Centre, both in Washington, DC. Pellegrino advocated that the *wounded humanity* of patients be seen and understood by the medical profession. He recognised four major losses for the humanity of those who fall ill: the loss of freedom of action; the loss of freedom to make rational choices; the loss of freedom from the power of others, and the loss of a sense of the integrity of the self.[1] His teachings have exerted a world-wide influence on the practice of medicine and his insights are helpful for the exploration of the experiences of loss and trauma in women with chronic invisible illnesses.

Philosopher Hugo Engelhardt explained in an article in the *Journal of Medicine and Philosophy* (1990) 'from the beginning of this century into the early seventies, the humanities and medicine had become progressively estranged .... On the side of medicine, knowledge and power expanded so rapidly as to outpace the reflective capacities of the profession.'[2] The bias in favour of science at the expense of empathy with the patient has its origins in the Flexner Report which had been published in 1910 under the aegis of the Carnegie Foundation.

## The Flexner Report

In an article in the *Journal of the American Medical Association (JAMA)*, in 2004, Andrew H. Beck of Stanford University investigated the roots of the problem which gave rise to the inauguration of medical humanities in the USA. Beck explained how, in the early years of the twentieth century, medical training had been highly variable and inadequate.

> Some doctors were trained through an apprenticeship system, in which they worked alongside a local general practitioner. Others were given courses of lectures from physicians who owned private colleges; more attended university and worked in

---

1    S. Spicker and R. Ratzan, 'Ars Medicina Et Conditio Humana Edmund D. Pellegrino, M. D., on His 70th Birthday', *Journal of Medicine and Philosophy* 15, no. 3 (1 June 1990): 327, <https://doi.org/10.1093/jmp/15.3.327>.

2    H. Engelhardt, 'The Birth of the Medical Humanities and the Rebirth of the Philosophy of Medicine: The Vision of Edmund D. Pellegrino', *Journal of Medicine and Philosophy* 15, no. 3 (1 June 1990): 237–41, <https://doi.org/10.1093/jmp/15.3.237>.

hospitals to gain experience. In those days doctors were taught diverse types of medicine, 'scientific, osteopathic, homeopathic, chiropractic, eclectic, physiomedical, botanical and Thomsonian'.[3]

To resolve the issue of non-standardised training, the American Medical Association (AMA) began campaigning in 1904 for more scientific rigour in the training of medical doctors and set about re-structuring medical education. In 1909, education reformer Abraham Flexner (1866–1959) was commissioned, with funding from the Carnegie Foundation, to carry out research on how medical education could be improved. An article in *JAMA* in 2010, marking the centenary of the Report, portrayed a picture of Flexner's labours more than a century earlier:

> For 16 months, from January 1909 through April 1910, Abraham Flexner crisscrossed North America via train, horse and buggy, and the occasional Ford flivver. Along the way he visited 98 cities and made 174 separate inspections of 155 medical schools. In April 1909 alone, he surveyed some 30 schools in 12 cities.[4]

The Flexner Report *Medical Education in the United States and Canada*[5] constituted a stinging attack on medical training in North America. The scathing tone of the Report was captured in Flexner's critique of the California Medical College:

> Its so called equipment is dirty and disorderly beyond description. Its outfit in anatomy consists of a small box of bones and the few dried up filthy fragments of a single cadaver ... the school is a disgrace to the state whose laws permit its existence.[6]

3    A. Beck, 'The Flexner Report and the Standardization of American Medical Education', *JAMA: The Journal of the American Medical Association* 291, no. 17 (5 May 2004): 2139–40, <https://doi.org/10.1001/jama.291.17.2139>.

4    H. Markel, 'Abraham Flexner and His Remarkable Report on Medical Education: A Century Later', *JAMA: The Journal of the American Medical Association* 303, no. 9 (2 March 2010): 888–90, <https://doi.org/10.1001/jama.2010.225>.

5    A. Flexner, 'Medical Education in the United States and Canada' (New York: The Carnegie Foundation, 1910), <http://archive.carnegiefoundation.org/pdfs/elibrary/Carnegie_Flexner_Report.pdf>.

6    H. Pritchett and A. Flexner, *Medical Education in the United States and Canada: A Report to the Carnegie Foundation for the Advancement of Teaching*, Bulletin (Carnegie

Flexner's Report resulted in reforms in medical training throughout the USA which still form the basis of the training of medical doctors today. Flexner insisted on higher standards of education for those entering medical colleges, and graduating from them. He advocated that the medical schools be properly equipped and linked to high standard teaching hospitals. He also espoused the principle that the medical colleges should adhere to mainstream science, grounded in physiology and biochemistry. Many of the medical colleges involved in his study were later closed down.

Flexner defined the purpose of medicine as the attempt to fight disease. The application of scientific methods to the investigation and control of disease has paid dividends. However, the damaging consequences of Flexner's Report for the human aspect of medicine were highlighted in an article by two medical doctors, Samir Johna and Simi Rahman, in 2011 in *Permanente*, a journal of the medical humanities: 'But we know that patients are not just bodies, organs, and tissues. They live meaning-centred lives, and they have complicated emotional and historical relationships with their bodies.' Johna and Rahman, both advocates of a more patient-centred and compassion-rich approach, went on to say, 'Flexner's vision of medical education created physicians richly sophisticated in biologic variables and interventions, but all too often they lost touch with the human aspects of health care and the basic tenets of clinical encounters with their patients.'[7] A growing awareness of the abyss that was continuing to widen in medicine led to a number of concerned professionals coming together in the USA to find a solution.

---

Foundation for the Advancement of Teaching); No. 4. (New York City: [Carnegie Foundation for the Advancement of Teaching], 1910), 190, <http://nrs.harvard.edu/urn-3:HMS.COUNT:1181036>.

7    S. Johna and S. Rahman, 'Humanity before Science: Narrative Medicine, Clinical Practice, and Medical Education', *The Permanente Journal* 15, no. 4 (2011): 92–4.

## Bridging the Gap between Doctor and Patient

The *Society for Health and Human Values* was established in Philadelphia in 1969 by medical academic administrators and scholars with the aim of identifying and resolving problems caused by the rapid advances of science in medicine. These pioneers set up the *Institute of Human Values in Medicine* in 1971, in New York, with Edmund Pellegrino as chairman. In a series of meetings throughout the 1970s, the Institute began to create medical humanities and work out a way of incorporating the concept in medical education: 'It initiated a program of visits to campuses by persons with competence in the humanities and in medicine to advise faculty on ways of introducing humanities into the curriculum'.[8]

Right throughout the 1970s, attempts were made to bridge the gap between science and human experience; courses on social sciences and humanities were introduced in many of the medical schools in the USA. The aim was to educate more humane physicians.[9] Currently most of the faculties of medicine in the USA have medical humanities programmes; the movement has spread globally.

The British Medical Journal and the Institute of Medical Ethics co-own a specialist online publication titled *Medical Humanities*, which was launched in 2000. The publication reflects the broad span of interest of this field. This international, peer-reviewed journal features articles 'relevant to the delivery of healthcare, the formulation of public health policy, the experience of being ill and of caring for those who are ill, as well as case conferences, educational case studies, book, film, and art reviews, editorials, correspondence, news and notes'.[10]

The medical humanities website of the New York University (NYU) School of Medicine claims that the humanities provide unique insight into

8   A. Jonsen, *The Birth of Bioethics* (New York: Oxford University Press, 2003), 25.
9   R. Puustinen, M. Leiman, and A. Viljanen, 'Medicine and the Humanities – Theoretical and Methodological Issues', *Medical Humanities* 29, no. 2 (1 December 2003): 77–80, <https://doi.org/10.1136/mh.29.2.77>.
10  <http://mh.bmj.com/site/about/>. Accessed 3 June 2015.

the human condition and facilitate an understanding of human suffering in a more than scientific way:

> Attention to literature and the arts helps to develop and nurture skills of observation, analysis, empathy, and self-reflection – skills that are essential for humane healthcare. The social sciences help us to understand how bioscience and medicine take place within cultural and social contexts and how culture interacts with the individual experience of illness and the way healthcare is practiced.[11]

In order to set the scene for the type of reading of the medical histories of those interviewed in this research, a fuller exploration of the humanities turn in medicine will be offered here. Arthur Kleinman and Rita Charon, American medical doctors and professors, are eminent proponents of a more humane approach to medicine. They have a specific interest in an interdisciplinary discourse in medical settings and are advocates of *narrative medicine*.

---

11    <http://medhum.med.nyu.edu/about>. Accessed 31 May 2015.

# Contemporary Medical Humanitarians Respond

## Arthur Kleinman: Illness and Anthropology

Harvard professor Arthur Kleinman has gained international prominence as a medical anthropologist. A distinguished humanitarian, he has campaigned for most of his career for the inclusion of greater morality in medicine. His anthropological interests led him to China to study the differences between the views of the Chinese people and the American people on issues around illness, thus enabling him to position narratives of illness in the context of social construction and culture.

Kleinman's interest in interdisciplinary scholarship became evident in his early years at Stanford University, between 1962 and 1967, where he graduated initially in the social sciences and subsequently in medicine. In 1974 he obtained a Master's degree in social anthropology at Yale University. This wide range of interests manifested in his later work as a doctor, teacher and author, where he consistently emphasised the need for a broad context for medicine, disease and diagnosis.

Kleinman has fostered a deep interest in chronic illness and spent much of his career since 1969 conducting ethnographic studies in China examining how people experience illness and tell their stories. During his time there, he developed a deep respect for Confucianism, which for many centuries had influenced moral and philosophical thought in China. Confucian philosophy affords importance to ethics, civilised behaviour, decency, morality, the family and the idea of becoming more human as we go through life. Kleinman has argued that the study of the narratives of illness has a lot to teach us about the human condition, and its engagement with suffering and death. Illness narratives teach us, he said, 'about how life problems are created, controlled, made meaningful'.[1]

Kleinman has emphasised the importance of distinguishing between the terms 'illness' and 'disease': Illness is what the patient experiences. Disease, on the other hand, is what the doctor diagnoses: 'The practitioner reconfigures the patient's and family's illness problems as narrow technical issues, disease problems'.[2] Doctors need to understand, he emphasised, that human problems cannot be reduced to simplistic formulas and stereotyped manipulations that treat patients and their families as if they were overly rational mannequins. The doctor's diagnosis is a reduction of the experience of the patient. He argued, however, that it is possible to craft a clinical method that is neither reductionist nor mechanistic. For the purpose of this research, Kleinman's approach is of particular interest – many with invisible illnesses experience distress when their descriptions of their physical illness are not substantiated by the results of their medical examinations.

Kleinman is a prolific writer who has authored many works in the fields of medical anthropology, cross-cultural psychiatry, public health, chronic illness and disability. This research has selected themes from his writings which will help to illuminate the experiences of women with chronic invisible illnesses to be presented later in this study. These themes include: life-altering illness and culture; neurasthenia in China; illness versus disease; the Western view of mental illness versus the anthropologist's findings, and stigma.

Kleinman's first major work *Patients and Healers in the Context of Culture* (1980) was authored following extensive research into the treatment of disease in Taiwan. The book presented his theoretical framework of how to study the relationships between medicine and psychiatry, as well as culture and psychiatry. It was the latter area of interest that led him to study medical and psychiatric anthropology.[3] He wished to explore the

---

1    A. Kleinman, *The Illness Narratives: Suffering, Healing, And The Human Condition* (New York: Basic Books, 1989), xiii.
2    Ibid., 228.
3    A. Kleinman, *Patients and Healers in the Context of Culture: An Exploration of the Borderland between Anthropology, Medicine, and Psychiatry* (Berkeley: University of California Press, 1980), 19.

ways in which differing cultural views on sickness and treatment affect clinical communication between patient, family and practitioners. He was also interested in determining 'culture-specific and universal characteristics of the healing process'.[4]

*Patients and Healers in the Context of Culture* encouraged students of medicine and doctors to broaden their horizons so as to see culture as an important variable in clinical practice and to encourage anthropologists to see culture as part of medicine rather than the other way around. Kleinman documented narratives and case studies from his fieldwork in Taiwan. His study investigated the myriad of medical services available in Taiwan, including shamans (tang-ki), oracles, bone-setters, classical Chinese medicine, and Western medicine. He painted a picture of the background assumptions around health care in Taiwan, for example that medicine was a family affair and thus private consultations with doctors were considered unacceptable.

Mental illness, Kleinman found, was considered shameful in Taiwan, and consequently mental distress tended to become somatised. These findings illuminate the issue of how illness is culturally constructed. Kleinman notes that his observations 'forced me to recognise, not just that the biomedical model was freighted with Western cultural assumptions and saturated with a particular theoretical and value orientation, but that it had no means for taking into account patient and lay perspectives'.[5] The book could be criticised for claiming to present a cross-cultural study of illness, when in reality it focused on only two cultures, that of Taiwan and, to a lesser degree, Boston. Nevertheless, by presenting the reader with the vast array of the choice of cures available in Taiwan, and that country's culturally specific attitudes towards illness, his argument that the Western perspectives are limited carries weight.

This publication was followed in 1986 by another work on the theme of illness perspectives in Chinese culture. Based on research carried out by Kleinman in the early 1980s in the Hunan Medical University in China, *Social Origins of Disease: Depression, Neurasthenia, and Pain in modern*

4    Ibid., 18.
5    Ibid., 18.

*China* presents an attempt to understand the place of neurasthenia in modern China and the relationship of neurasthenia to depression. The term *neurasthenia* had been popularised by an American neurologist, Dr George Beard, around 1869. Webster's 1913 dictionary located the provenance of the word in ancient Greek and proffered a definition of 'a condition of nervous debility supposed to be dependent on impairment of the spinal cord'.[6] Neurasthenia was characterised by a range of symptoms which included weakness, exhaustion not cured by sleep, aches and pains, dizziness and gastrointestinal upsets. It is of particular interest to this research that neurasthenia is sometimes offered by researchers of the history of ME/CFS as an example of an illness with similar symptoms and characteristics. In her popular narrative of her own experience with the illness, American poet and author, Dorothy Wall, provides an interesting account of the way in which 'putting these distant cousins into the same room can open an intriguing conversation ... about the deficiencies and the limits of the medical system these patients confront'.[7]

Kleinman found that in China neurasthenia represented, together with schizophrenia, the most common diagnosis given to psychiatric outpatients. However, in Europe and North America, neurasthenia gradually disappeared from diagnostic practice between the 1930s and 1960s.[8] In contrast to North America where the most common diagnosis for psychiatric outpatients is

6    Webster's Dictionary, 'Webster's Revised Unabridged Dictionary (1913) – The ARTFL Project', 1913, <http://machaut.uchicago.edu/?resource=Webster%27s&word=neurasthenia&use1913=on>. Accessed 12 September 2015.

7    D. Wall, *Encounters with the Invisible: Unseen Illness, Controversy, and Chronic Fatigue Syndrome* (Dallas, TX: Southern Methodist University Press, 2005), 95. Although it is 'popular' in genre, this review of the history, science and politics of the illness has a commendation on its book-cover by the director of the medical humanities programme at the Feinberg School of Medicine in Chicago.

8    M. L. Schäfer, 'On the history of the concept neurasthenia and its modern variants chronic-fatigue-syndrome, fibromyalgia and multiple chemical sensitivities', *Fortschritte Der Neurologie-Psychiatrie* 70, no. 11 (November 2002): 570–82, <https://doi.org/10.1055/s-2002-35174>.

depression, the diagnosis of depression was hardly ever used in China.[9] Kleinman found that it was more acceptable in China to be labelled with neurasthenia than to have the diagnosis of mental illness of any sort, which would lead to total alienation not just of the individual sufferer but also of the family. The Cultural Revolution which started in China in 1966 brought persecution for millions of people, including the mentally ill. The Chinese governor, Chairman Mao Zedong (1893–1976), declared that depression and other mental illnesses were synonymous with wrong political thinking. Everyone was expected to be energetic and participative in society. In this political context, neurasthenia constituted a more acceptable and a safer diagnosis.

Traditional Chinese medicine views the syndrome of physical weakness and fatigue, accompanied by low mood, as a symptom of blocked *chi* (energy), therefore neurasthenia had a comfortable home in that Chinese medicine worldview. Kleinman found that, unlike in Western societies, neurasthenia can justify early retirement for those who suffer from it. Many people with ME find consolation and affirmation when they visit an acupuncturist or Chinese herbalist, as the practitioner acknowledges the condition without an overlay of the guilt induced in Western medicine.

Of 100 people researched who had been diagnosed with neurasthenia in China, Kleinman found that by American criteria, ninety-three would be diagnosed with depression, and eighty-seven of those with a major depressive disorder. He proceeded to give an historical account of neurasthenia and depression in China and in the West, sketching how the term came into China in colonial times, and subsequently went into disuse in the West. These themes formed the basis of a wide-ranging discussion in the book on the various ways in which illness conditions are configured in different social and cultural backgrounds.

9   A. Kleinman, 'Review: Social Origins of Distress and Disease: Depression, Neurasthenia and Pain in Modern China', *Current Anthropology*, 5, 27, no. 5 (1 December 1986): 499–509.

In 1988 Kleinman conducted collaborative narrative research on CFS in the USA with Norma Ware,[10] now associate professor at the Department of Global Health at Harvard Medical School. This was building on the research carried out earlier on neurasthenia in China. Fifty patients with CFS were interviewed in the USA using an approach similar to that used by Kleinman and Kleinman in China. They noted that 80 per cent of the subjects with CFS were female. The study examined the way in which symptoms are influenced by the social world, and, in turn, illness experience bears influence on society, and ways in which illness can act as a force for transformation in the individual's world, and the worlds of those around them. Somatic experience is both created by and creates culture throughout the social course of illness. The authors critique the way in which culture has relatively rarely been incorporated in biomedical research.

Ware and Kleinman found that sufferers of CFS in the USA had been leading lives of intense activity before the onset of the illness. Those who were employed devoted sixty, seventy or even eighty hours a week to their jobs. Some of the women also had responsibilities, for example, rearing their children, studying, or caring for a parent. A desire for accomplishment and success, combined with setting high personal performance standards, 'impelled these individuals always to try harder, go further, in an attempt to meet the expectations that they had set for themselves at work, at home and at school.'[11] Whereas in China the social forces that shaped the somatic experience of neurasthenia included political turmoil and terror, in America CFS reflected the conflicting demands and pressures, on women in particular.

Kleinman discussed the cultural construction of illness in 1989 in *The Illness Narratives: Suffering, Healing and the Human Condition;* however, in this instance *culture* can simply mean the values and habits prevailing in a family or community: 'Paradoxical as it sounds, then, there are normal ways of being ill (ways that our society regards as appropriate) as

---

10   N. C. Ware and A. Kleinman, 'Culture and Somatic Experience: The Social Course of Illness in Neurasthenia and Chronic Fatigue Syndrome', *Psychosomatic Medicine* 54, no. 5 (October 1992): 546–60.

11   Ibid., 551.

well as anomalous ways'.[12] In the book, he also addressed the issue of the dichotomy between the technological advances which have been made in medicine and the actual treatment of those who are sick, handicapped or dying. Kleinman's observations are relevant to the research topic and help illuminate the circumstances and experiences of women with illnesses who, because of cultural biases, experience not being believed by doctors.

In *The Illness Narratives*, Kleinman also argued for a distinction that needs to be made between the terms *disease* and *illness*, that is, the patient's experience of illness versus the doctor's attention to disease.[13] He emphasised the importance of listening to patients' narratives and taking into account patients' emotions, not just as a peripheral exercise but as a central component to care. In summary, he proposed that medical practitioners ought to focus on the illness of the patient, rather than the disease. He recommended that mini-ethnographies be undertaken of chronically ill people and he maintained that students of medicine need to know how to interpret the patients' narratives as well as the illness experience. Kleinman lamented that medical training 'inculcates values and behaviours that are antithetical to the humane care of patients'.[14]

*A Passion for Society: How We Think about Human Suffering*, Kleinman's collaborative work with sociologist Iain Wilkinson, criticises social science for moving away from a key aspiration of the founders which was to improve people's lives.[15] Social science has lost its way in this regard. They argue that it is no longer tenable for social science to be dispassionate and that it needs to engage in the practice of caregiving. The authors assert a commitment to 'a social research practice that is sustained not so much by a quest for academic recognition but more by a moral concern to be actively involved

---

12  Kleinman, *The Illness Narratives*, 5.

13  Ibid.

14  Ibid., 257.

15  I. Wilkinson and A. Kleinman, *A Passion for Society: How We Think about Human Suffering*, California Series in Public Anthropology; 35 (Oakland: University of California Press, 2016), <http://nrs.harvard.edu/urn-3:hul. ebook:EBSCO_9780520962408>.

in the creation of humane forms of society'.[16] Again, Kleinman understands the power of human suffering to shatter one's foundations, and to bring about losses of roles, identities and relationships. On the optimistic side, the authors recognise the way in which 'the brute force of suffering works on us so that we attend with heightened alertness and alarm to the ways in which our lives are marked by social circumstance'.[17]

Kleinman drew on his training as an anthropologist in his application of the mini-ethnography to the care of the chronically ill. His insights have influenced the manner in which the interviews were conducted and analysed for this study. Like the anthropologist, the ethnographer-doctor figuratively visits a foreign land, that of the ill person, learning the language and describing the environment. She tries to see things from the native's point of view and tries to enter the experiential world of the native, or chronically ill person in this case. This experiential phenomenology is the entrée into the world of the sick, and the families who care for them.[18] The task of gathering data for the mini-ethnography is in itself often psychotherapeutic for the patient.

Kleinman expressed disquiet that an anthropological approach to psychiatry was considered marginal in his profession and asked, 'why should so strongly Western oriented a discipline regard cross cultural research among the more than 80 per cent of the world's people who inhabit non-Western societies as marginal?'[19] He considered how a diagnosis is made, and how so-called disorders are conceptualised in different cultures. This theme was introduced in a book which he co-authored with Byron Good in 1986 entitled *Culture and Depression: Studies in Anthropology and Cross-cultural Psychiatry of Affect and Disorder*. In the book he provided a fascinating overview of the conceptualisation of depression in different cultures.

For Buddhists, depression could be considered the first step on the road to salvation, for Shi'ite Muslims in Iran, depression could, in certain

---

16    Ibid., 22.
17    Ibid., 9.
18    Kleinman, *The Illness Narratives*, 233.
19    A. Kleinman, *Rethinking Psychiatry: From Cultural Category to Personal Experience*,
      1st edn (New York: Free Press, 1991), xii.

circumstances, be seen as a 'marker of depth and understanding of a person'.[20] The Kaluli of Papua New Guinea, he noted, value dramatic expressions of sadness. Later, his 1991 publication, *Rethinking Psychiatry*, examined the effectiveness of the clinical tools of psychiatry compared with the healing tools of other non-Western cultures. This work concluded with thoughts on how psychiatry could interact with the social sciences, to foster once again a more humane approach towards mental illness. Overall the book's strength lies in its recognition of the limitations of some traditional diagnostic categories and offers the possibility of a conceptualisation of mental illness as not merely residing within the person but also having the possibility of being understood as a social phenomenon.

Kleinman believes that chronic illness by definition cannot be cured, that even searching for a cure is a dangerous exercise that serves neither the patient nor the doctor. The popular idea that all diseases can be cured creates frustration for patients and carers. He has argued that the primary goal of treatment should be the reduction of disablement over the long term course of the illness.[21]

Kleinman affirms the right of chronically ill persons to become experts on their illnesses and to develop skills to treat themselves.[22] These sentiments on chronic illness are pertinent for those with ME and other invisible illnesses. He is acutely aware of the shame and stigma surrounding chronic illness, citing Erving Goffman (1922–1982), the Canadian sociologist whose book entitled *Stigma: Notes on the Management of Spoiled Identity* expressed sentiments which ring true for people with chronic invisible illnesses. The word *stigma* derives from Greek and means to mark or brand: 'The signs were cut or burnt into the body and advertised that the bearer was a slave, a criminal or a traitor – a blemished person, ritually

---

20   A. Kleinman and B. Good, *Culture and Depression: Studies in the Anthropology and Cross-Cultural Psychiatry of Affect and Disorder* (Oakland: University of California Press, 1986), 3.

21   Kleinman, *The Illness Narratives*, 229.

22   Ibid., 261.

polluted, to be avoided, especially in public places'.[23],[24] Goffman's analysis of stigma and the ways in which people's identities get spoiled have grown into stigma theory, which is given significant attention in disability studies. His main focus was ways in which social hierarchies are built, maintained and given legitimacy through the dynamics of face-to-face interaction.[25] Goffman argued that there is a basic pressure on individuals to maintain a positive self-image, to 'maintain face'. Scambler and Hopkins delineated two kinds of stigma: 'felt stigma' refers to a fear of being stigmatised, and 'enacted stigma' pertains to actual discrimination by others. In the literature on chronic pain and contested illnesses in general, stigma features prominently. An extensive literature search conducted by Newton et al. on the manner in which those with chronic pain may experience disbelief in relation to their pain yielded stigma as a primary theme.[26]

The following passage from Kleinman is pertinent to many people with invisible or contested illnesses; they experience illness, but the disbelief of the medical profession in their illness leads to their social stigmatisation:

> In stigmatised disorders, the stigma can begin with the societal reaction to the condition: that is to say a person so labeled is shunned, derided, disconfirmed, and degraded by those around him ... eventually the stigmatised person comes to expect such reactions, to anticipate them before they occur or even when they don't occur. By that stage, he has thoroughly internalised the stigma in a deep sense of shame and spoiled identity. His behaviour then becomes shaped by his negative self-perception.[27]

Here Kleinman alerts his readers to the power of society to determine where the boundary lies in relation to what is an acceptable illness versus an unacceptable illness.

23    E. Goffman, *Stigma: Notes on the Management of Spoiled Identity* (New York: Touchstone, 1986), 1.

24    Kleinman, *The Illness Narratives*, 158.

25    A. J. Treviño, *Goffman's Legacy* (Lanham, MD: Rowman & Littlefield, 2003), 105.

26    Benjamin J. Newton et al., 'A Narrative Review of the Impact of Disbelief in Chronic Pain', *Pain Management Nursing* 14, no. 3 (September 2013): 161–71, <https://doi.org/10.1016/j.pmn.2010.09.001>.

27    Kleinman, *The Illness Narratives*, 160.

# Rita Charon: Deep Listening to the Patient's Narrative

A pioneer in the joint field of medicine and the humanities, Rita Charon was appointed Professor of Clinical Medicine at the College of Physicians and Surgeons of Columbia University in New York in 2001. She had been teaching at the college since 1982 and founded its programme in *narrative medicine*. Charon calls her field *narrative medicine*, though she acknowledges its roots are a blend of biopsychosocial medicine, primary care, the medical humanities and patient-centred medicine.[28] She also acknowledges Dr Michael Balint as one of the progenitors of narrative medicine.[29] Balint was a psychoanalyst who set up a forum in the UK in 1950 for medical doctors to learn about the psychological dynamics involved in doctor-patient relationships. Her work is of particular interest here because she affirms the skill of being able to be present attentively with a patient, in a manner which facilitates the patient to tell her story and she also acknowledges the therapeutic value of narrative. Furthermore, Charon endeavours, by educating medical students in English literature, to ensure that future doctors acquire a capacity to listen to the deeper dimensions of the stories they hear.

In her first year as a medical student in 1974, Charon learned about the importance of listening attentively to the patients and hearing their stories with presence and respect. In this regard, she was highly influenced by her teacher and mentor at Harvard, Elliott Mishler. A social psychologist and a sociolinguist, Mishler had carried out important and influential work on the study of doctor-patient communication.[30]

As a trainee in internal medicine at the Residency Program in Social Medicine at Montefiore Hospital in New York after her graduation in 1978, Charon listened intently to the narratives of her patients. Following

28　R. Charon, *Narrative Medicine: Honoring the Stories of Illness* (Oxford ; New York: Oxford University Press, 2006), 6.

29　P. Rudnytsky and R. Charon, *Psychoanalysis and Narrative Medicine* (New York: SUNY Press, 2008), 3.

30　E. Mishler, *The Discourse of Medicine: Dialectics of Medical Interviews* (New York: Ablex Publishing, 1985).

a patient interview, she wrote up what she felt the patient had told her. The text was then presented to the patient, asking if this was a true representation of the patient's story. The patient was free to add or change anything the doctor had written. In 1981, Charon carried this practice of narrative medicine into Columbia University where she started out as a fellow in general medicine, and then progressed to teacher of clinical medicine at Columbia's College of Physicians. In 2001 she was promoted to professor.

Charon studied English literature, in parallel to her work, at Columbia University and obtained an MA in English Literature in 1990. This was followed by a PhD on the work of Henry James and the use of literary methods in understanding the texts and work of medicine. Her motivation was to use narrative skills in order to become a better doctor:

> I could listen to what my patients tell me with a greater ability to follow the narrative thread of their story, to recognize the governing images and metaphors, to adopt the patients' or family members' points of view, to identify the sub-texts present in all stories, to interpret one story in the light of others told by the same teller. Moreover, the better I was as 'reader' of what my patients told me, the more deeply moved I myself was by their predicament, making more of myself available to patients as I tried to help.[31]

Rita Charon has written extensively on ethics in medical practice, the doctor-patient relationship, empathy, and narrative competence. However, for the purposes of this study of narratives of women with chronic ill-health, some of her relevant publications on the topic of narrative in relation to medical ethics and in relation to illness and to psychoanalysis were deemed to be of particular importance.

Published in 2002, *Stories Matter: The Role of Narrative in Medical Ethics* was co-edited by Rita Charon and Professor Martha Montello who was also at the forefront of the narrative medicine movement. The book developed a theme about narrative in the context of ethical medicine

---

31    R. Charon, 'LitSite Alaska | Perspectives', 2000, <http://www.litsite.org/index. cfm?section=Narrative-and-Healing&page=Perspectives&viewpost=2&Conten tId=985>. Accessed 26 May 2011.

which Charon had flagged in 1996 in the *Journal of Ethical Philosophy*.[32] She discussed the significance of narrative for the field of medical ethics and how literature actually works in helping doctors in the practice of ethical medicine. She argued, citing five case studies, that when doctors apply literary methods in analysing the narratives of patients, doctors were enabled to practise in a wide range of ethically challenging contexts. The book was compiled against a background debate ongoing in the medical ethics establishment around 'principlism' versus 'narrative' approaches. Principlism is a system of ethics based on four principles: autonomy (free will); beneficence (to do good); non-maleficence (to do no harm), and justice (the social distribution of benefits and burdens). The contributors to the book were clear that the principlist approach did not necessarily need to be abandoned, but that narrative methods needed to be incorporated. The book assembled twenty-three bioethicists and literary theorists who were experts in their field. Each one made a case for the use of narrative in bioethics.

One of the contributors, Richard Martinez, explained: 'Narrative methods help us to listen and see with intensified accuracy and reach – a hermeneutic stethoscope of a sort.'[33] Jerome Bruner, psychologist, contributed a discussion on the Aristotelian concept of *peripeteia* meaning the unexpected incident in life or in the narrative that changes everything: 'We start out with some canonical expectancies of what the world is like, how things are going to be, and then all of a sudden things happen differently ... all of a sudden, you get cancer or the wife leaves you.'[34] Doctors often have to deliver the peripeteia, the news that alters the expected and that in time becomes adapted into the narrative of the patient.

The book stressed the importance for physicians to be trained in *close listening* to the narratives of the patients in order to be able to make ethical

32   R. Charon et al., 'Literature and Ethical Medicine: Five Cases from Common Practice', *The Journal of Medicine and Philosophy* 21 (1996): 243–65.

33   R. Charon and M. Montello, *Stories Matter: The Role of Narrative in Medical Ethics*, 1st edn (New York: Routledge, 2002), 131.

34   Ibid., 4.

decisions. It provided guidelines and conceptual foundations for practitioners in medical ethics issues.

In her book *Narrative Medicine, Honouring the Stories of Illness*, published in 2006, Charon introduced the conceptual principles which underpin narrative medicine and illustrated how narrative methods can be used in clinical practice. Medicine, she has argued, has made great progress but often lacks empathy. She posited that the modern health care system could become 'more effective than it has been in treating disease by recognising and respecting those afflicted with it and in nourishing those who care for the sick'.[35] Charon discussed the notion of the self being the caregiver's most powerful therapeutic instrument, and its consequent implication that health care professionals have to work towards self-awareness.

Narratology is a useful tool to this end. Charon considers it crucial not just for understanding the patient but also for gaining self-awareness; she wrote that narratology was often the 'silent partner to human beings as they make and mark meaning, coping with the contingencies of moral and mental life'.[36] She pointed out how medicine lagged behind other disciplines saying, 'A narrative shift has taken place across ... many fields of human learning, challenging scholars and practitioners from religious studies to psychoanalysis to police work to concentrate not just on the facts, but on the situations in which the facts are told'.[37] Her theories on the power of narrative, and on the self as a therapeutic instrument, will help to illuminate the frankness of the participants of the research.

Charon offered a vision of listening with presence, 'heads of the teller and the listener are bowed over the suffering that happened in an attempt to interpret it and understand it'.[38] This attentive listening could enable patients to come out of their solitude in sickness; in support, she quotes John Donne (1572–1631), 'as sickenesse is the greatest misery, so the greatest misery of sickenesse is *solitude*'.[39]

---

35    Charon, *Narrative Medicine*, 4.
36    Ibid., 40.
37    Ibid., 11.
38    Ibid., 12.
39    J. Donne, *The Works of John Donne* (J. W. Parker, 1839), 513.

Charon wrote at length about the chasm between the healthy doctor and the sick patient, one example of the many divides in medical practice; others exist between doctors and nurses, social workers and psychiatrists, home-care nurses and hospital nurses, for example. Narrative, she felt, could bridge this gap. However, the gap between the sick and the well is 'capricious, unpredictable, sometimes reversible, but in the end irrevocable'.[40] She argued that there exists a divide between doctor and patient in relation to their views about death and illness. Doctors see illness as a biological phenomenon to be treated, for the patient the illness is seen within the frame and scope of their entire lives. Echoing Kleinman,[41] she believed there was a conflict between what the doctor sees as the cause of the disease, and the patient's view. The emotions of shame, blame and fear divide doctor and patient, in that the patient frequently carries these emotions and the doctor does not. Charon's work on the chasms between the doctor and the patient, the sick and the well, will be helpful in illuminating issues raised in the interviews conducted for this study.

*Narrative Medicine* presented Charon's model of the *parallel chart*, a method in which Charon's students of medicine are trained at Columbia University. Alongside writing up a clinical chart, students are asked to draw up a 'parallel chart'. In this reflexive record, the student is required to journal what she thought of the patient, what impact in personal terms the patient had on her. If the patient reminded her of her grandmother and annoyed her, she would write this down, for example. Charon advocates a more humane approach to medicine and asserts that the telling of narratives of pain and suffering is crucial for the recovery of the patient. Narrating the story helps the patient to frame her experience so she is not dominated by it. Charon considered the act of telling one's story a cry for affirmation and a way to create a sense of self.

Her treatise on patient narratives, however, omits any discussion on how women may experience illness in ways which are different to the experiences of men, with the exception of a footnote to the fourth chapter in *Narrative Medicine*. Here, Charon signposted a paucity of research

40   Charon, *Narrative Medicine*, 21.
41   Kleinman, *The Illness Narratives*, 5.

on gender differences in narratives of illness: 'Although a comparison of women's pathographies with men's pathographies has not been undertaken, one wonders how these gendered differences in telling of the self would maintain when the self is ill.'

Elsewhere, Charon has spoken out strongly against gender injustice in medicine. In a preface to *Gendered Scripts and Medicine* (2010), a publication which drew on literature and the arts to investigate the effects of gender stereotypes in shaping the way medicine has been practised and perceived throughout the ages, Charon criticised gender inequality in the medical profession:

> Medicine can hardly be bested as an arena in which to inspect gender injustice. The very terms of engagement of feminist studies arose from the medical sphere – the panoptic gaze, the clinical objectification, the machine of power. As the *ur*-narrative of women's struggles against male-dominated systems of power, medical struggles repeat and reproduce the consequences of the dominant discourse over enforced silence, of the knot of knowledge and power against ignorance and weakness, and of the advantage that can be taken of human need.[42]

Charon's advocacy of narrative medicine provides validation for the narrative approach adopted in the methodology of the research presented here. These insights into gender injustice in the medical world will also illuminate the narratives of women, to be presented later, who have felt their illness experiences being negated in a medical context. She has advocated narrative training not just for doctors but ultimately for anyone working near sick people, including ward clerks and transport workers. Her ideals may appear unrealistic for the practice of medicine with its inherent time pressures and limited resources. Charon has stated that she spends approximately an hour with each patient in her practice in New York. She did not specify whether this practice is private or publicly funded. In the UK and in Ireland, under the current systems, a fraction of that time is available to GPs – rendering it difficult for narrative medicine to take hold in the

---

42   R. Charon, 'Preface', in *Gender Scripts in Medicine and Narrative*, eds M. Block and A. Laflen (Newcastle upon Tyne, 2010), xiv–xviii, <http://www.cambridgescholars. com/gender-scripts-in-medicine-and-narrative-16>. Accessed 4 August 2015.

GP's clinic. The website of the National Health Service (NHS) in the UK advises patients: 'Doctors spend an average of eight-10 minutes with each patient. Once you've got an appointment, plan ahead to make sure that you cover everything you want to discuss.'[43]

Such short consultation time is not conducive to narrative therapy, which requires patience and attentive listening. In situations where illnesses resist diagnosis in such a short period, brief consultation times are unsatisfactory for doctor and patient alike.

An article in the popular science magazine *Scientific American* (2005) reported that critics of Charon had argued that medical school time should be spent on scientific subjects rather than on narrative medicine. Nevertheless, the author, Marguerite Holloway, who is a Professor of Science Journalism at Columbia University, remarked on the way in which 'the students themselves are embracing this movement.'[44] Rita Charon's work has had a robust impact on the field of medical humanities. She has succeeded in gaining a place for narrative medicine on the curricula of many medical schools. Furthermore, in so doing, she has firmly introduced into medicine the idea that the self-aware listener is a powerful human tool for healing. This research features narratives of illness which were gathered using a method that has been influenced by Charon's assertion of the necessity for self-awareness on the part of the listener.

Charon extends her discussion on the limitations of the biomedical model in *Psychoanalysis and Narrative Medicine* which she co-edited in 2008 with Peter L. Rudnytsky, Professor of English at the University of Florida. In this publication Charon confronted, 'the undue simple mindedness of biomedicine' which, she said, has become 'paltry, limited, conceptually cramped, even as it takes pride in its dazzling complexity and daring.'[45] Charon added that, 'sick people are being abandoned left and right, not

43 &lt;http://www.nhs.uk/choiceintheNHS/Yourchoices/GPchoice/Pages/GPappointments.aspx&gt;. Accessed 4 June 2015.

44 M. Holloway, 'When Medicine Meets Literature: Scientific American', April 2005, &lt;http://www.scientificamerican.com/article.cfm?id=when-medicine-meets-liter&page=2&gt;. Accessed 6 February 2016.

45 Rudnytsky and Charon, *Psychoanalysis and Narrative Medicine*, 25.

because their doctors do not recognise their molecules but because they cannot apprehend their narratives.' As the title suggests, the book attempted to integrate psychoanalysis into the literature-medicine dyad in order to provide healing practitioners with insights from psychoanalytic theory on making the unconscious conscious.

Charon has diffidently stated that she has merely re-introduced into medicine what had been there before, a respect for narrative practices because 'the medicine of Hippocrates, Galen, Sydenham, Chekhov, Blackwell, Freud, and William Carlos Williams had certainly been nourished by them in the past'.[46] Like Kleinman, she observed the gulf between doctor and patient. Her solution, narrative medicine, is her lasting contribution to the medical humanities.

46    R. Charon, 'The Self-Telling Body', *Narrative Inquiry* 16, no. 1 (2006): 191–200.

# CHAPTER 3

# The Traumatic Nature of Chronic Invisible Illness: The Women's Voices

> It was totally traumatic to be transitioning into womanhood and transitioning into menstruation, and at the same time manifesting like a horrible illness, a horrible illness, because it took me 20 years to get a diagnosis, it took all of my 20s, and half of my 30s, before I finally got someone to figure out what was wrong with me.
>
> — ANGELA

Two overarching themes materialised from the research: the traumatic nature of chronic invisible illness, and the multifaceted nature of the spiritual awakenings that emerged over time in the research participants as a consequence. The magnitude of the trauma experienced on an ongoing basis was unexpected and disturbing. As a consequence, I conducted a search for literature which would illuminate the notion of trauma as a feature of chronic illness, but it turned up only a modest amount on the chronic, continuous trauma caused by the day to day experiences of living with protracted illness. I could find no literature whatsoever on trauma in cases of chronic invisible or contested illness. Whilst the majority of texts omit chronic illness as a cause or origin of trauma, there is some acknowledgement of chronic illness as a symptomatic expression of trauma, or post-traumatic stress disorder.[1] The dearth of study on the subject of illness as trauma sui generis has been acknowledged by Angelo Alonzo in an account on research he carried out as Professor of Sociology at Ohio

---

1    <http://www.ehospitalistnews.com/index.php?id=100713&tx_ttnews[tt_news]= 18623&cHash=3a09ea56a1d7834ed4afcb852fcb2b7f>. Accessed 28 April 2015.

State University. In the journal *Social Science and Medicine* (2000) he
acknowledged:

> Individuals experiencing chronic diseases have been studied with regard to depres-
> sion, anxiety and a variety of coping maladaptions, but negligible attention has been
> given to the PTSD potential of chronic disease over the life course. Yet, growing evi-
> dence suggests that the traumatogenic potential of chronic diseases ... may produce
> maladaptive illness coping over the life course.[2]

In her book *Trauma and Recovery*, Judith Herman, a medical doctor and
Professor of Psychiatry at Harvard Medical School, renowned for her distinctive contributions to the field of trauma theory, has presented an overview of the history of trauma theory which elucidates why chronic illness
as a source of chronic trauma does not feature in the literature. She argued
that our contemporary understanding of trauma is built upon a synthesis of
three historical lines of inquiry. Firstly, it arose from an investigation into
hysteria, a psychological disorder diagnosed in women, which emerged
from France in the late nineteenth century. The second wave of investigation into trauma took place after the First World War (1914–1918), as US
soldiers presented with shell shock.[3] This approach reached its fullness
after the war in Vietnam (1955–1975). More recently trauma came into
public awareness as the subject matter of sexual and domestic violence
against women, with the rise of feminism from the 1970s.[4]

Herman has argued that the reason trauma arose into public consciousness at these three times was that each phase of investigation was held and
supported by a strong political movement: 'In the absence of strong political
movements for human rights, the active process of bearing witness inevitably gives way to the active process of forgetting.'[5] Sufferers of all forms

---

2    A. Alonzo, 'The Experience of Chronic Illness and Post-Traumatic Stress Disorder:
     The Consequences of Cumulative Adversity', *Social Science & Medicine* 50, no. 10
     (2000): 1475–84.
3    A. Kardiner, *The Traumatic Neuroses of War* (Atlanta, GA: National Academies,
     1941).
4    J. Herman, *Trauma and Recovery* (New York: Basic Books, 1992), 7–32.
5    Ibid., 9.

of trauma need a supportive environment in order to be able to speak out about their pain. She contends that it is difficult to convey the reality of trauma in a way people will listen, and that women are especially susceptible to being unheard: 'When the victim is already devalued (a woman, a child), she may find that the most traumatic events of her life take place outside the realm of socially validated reality.'⁶ To date, no political or social movement has arisen to give validation to the trauma experiences emanating from chronic illness. The existential reality of sickness is suffered in silence and is given little media coverage. Herman's work challenges the silence which surrounds this journey through trauma.

The ongoing traumatic impact of life-altering illness was expressed by each of the participants. The narratives of the trauma had many diverse identifying features. Aspects of trauma were identified in relation to the early years of the illness as respondents endeavoured to sustain working or studying despite the illness. Other features included not being believed by the medical profession; not being believed by others as a consequence of not being believed by the medical profession; having one's physical illness equated to mental disability; hurtful comments; loss; the perpetual nature of trauma in chronic invisible illness.

Other features of trauma, for example the distress caused by poverty, relationship difficulties and sleep difficulties, have not been specifically addressed here. They are briefly mentioned and occurred throughout most of the narratives as an undercurrent. If there was more money, for example, the participants would have had better access to holistic treatments. Those themes were omitted from this section owing to space limitations and also because they are a feature of many illnesses whether invisible or visible. A decision was made to maintain focus as much as possible on the traumatic features associated with the invisible characteristic of the illnesses.

---

6    Ibid., 8.

## Introducing the Nine Women

| | |
|---|---|
| Mary Rose | In her mid-fifties, Mary Rose has been ill for twenty-five years. She was a secondary school teacher when her health problems began, in the aftermath of an operation for appendicitis. Her medical diagnoses include ME and Multiple Chemical Sensitivity. Chiefly house-bound, and living alone, she has been unable to work for twenty-five years. |
| Sally | Sally, who worked as an artist and art therapist, is in her mid-fifties. Her illness is ME, which began at age thirty-six. Sally walks with the aid of a cane and uses a mobility scooter. She lives alone in rural Ireland. She has written a book on her illness and has created sculptures depicting psychological growth in illness. |
| Angela | Angela, in her mid-fifties, became ill at the age of sixteen. Although extensive medical tests were carried out, she was told by doctors that there was nothing physical wrong with her. Finally, at the age of thirty-eight, twenty-two years after the onset of her illness, she emigrated to the USA where she was diagnosed with tuberculosis, and informed that TB had already destroyed her hip joints and her capacity to have children. Cured of TB now, Angela has other chronic health issues. She has a partner. |
| Alice | Alice, formerly an insurance clerk, is now in her mid-sixties. She has been ill since the age of twenty-four when she began to suffer chronic pain, but was not believed by doctors to have a physical illness. She was committed to a psychiatric hospital and misdiagnosed with anorexia nervosa. Five years into her illness, Alice was finally diagnosed and had surgery for a twisted bowel. She has never regained her health nor recovered from the trauma of the psychiatric treatment. Her diagnosis now is ME and Multiple Chemical Sensitivity. She is single. |

| | |
|---|---|
| Orla | Orla, a single woman in her mid-fifties, works one day a week in a government department in her town. Her health has fluctuated since the age of sixteen when she developed ME which necessitated long periods of absence from school. However, she did not obtain a diagnosis of ME until her early twenties. She also has had cancer. |
| Patricia | Patricia, who lives in a small town, is now in her mid-fifties. She worked as a public servant until she fell ill at twenty-seven with severe pain and other chronic health problems. She was unable to sustain working because of cognitive symptoms. |
| Rachel | Rachel, a mother in her sixties, struggled with working as a teacher while suffering from severe pain for many years before taking early retirement. She was diagnosed with fibromyalgia which was not considered justification for early retirement. Her doctors advised her to substitute 'depression' for fibromyalgia in her application forms for early retirement. |
| Sharon | Sharon, a potter who had her own business, became ill ten years prior to the interview, following a mosquito bite. She has been diagnosed with chronic Lyme disease by a specialist in New York. She said her greatest loss was not being able to mother her teenage daughters, who were sent to live with an aunt in England who could take care of them. Sharon lives alone in a rural town. |
| Julia | Julia, a former nurse, is in her seventies. She is married but has not been able to live in her home for twenty years due to severe electromagnetic sensitivity. She suffers from severe pain, illness and acoustic sensitivity when exposed to mobile phones or phone masts. Julia sleeps in different houses, with relatives and friends, depending on the strength of the mobile phone signals emanating from masts, which fluctuates. She was told by doctors that she |

had a mental illness until she consulted a doctor who had spent time in Germany and recognised her condition as a physical one. She campaigns on the issue of electromagnetic sensitivity.

## Sustaining Employment Despite Illness

Seven of the nine respondents related the traumatic impact of the physical difficulty of sustaining their occupation during the early years of the illness. They continued to work irrespective of ill-health because they had no diagnosis, and therefore were unable to benefit from 'leave of absence' due to sickness. One respondent, Orla, elucidated, 'If you don't have a diagnosis, you can't get a proper sick certificate, and if you don't have a proper cert you have to keep going to work.' In respect of the other two respondents, one of them, Julia, had taken a summer break with the intention of returning to work but fell ill and has been unable to return to work since. The ninth, Sharon, did not speak of struggling to sustain work despite illness in her narrative. The following themes distilled from the narratives portray the insidious nature of the traumatic experiences of participants with this issue.

## Continuing to Work Despite Illness

Mary Rose continued to teach despite poor health for five years before gaining a diagnosis. Sally struggled to work for two years until she was hospitalised. From age sixteen until diagnosed with tuberculosis at thirty-eight, Angela worked and studied intermittently. Alice endured working from age twenty-four until she lost her job at thirty-two due to taking excessive sick leave. Orla persisted to study from onset of her illness at sixteen and through university years. She worked as a teacher for one year after completing her studies; she was advised by her boss that she was too ill to work. Patricia tried to continue working from illness onset, at twenty-seven, but was unable to sustain her job in the public service. She altered to part-time teaching but was unable to sustain that either. Rachel took sick leave from teaching for seven months, returned to work but then took a year and a half off. She was unable to return to work the following year and then gave up trying.

This clearly reflects a prolonged struggle to sustain employment and education for an unwarranted period of time when participants were unfit and unwell. Absence of diagnosis resulted in participants continuing with their normal pre-illness occupations until an event such as hospitalisation, further debility, or dismissal by an employer forced them to leave. The struggle of the participants is palpable in the summaries outlined above.

Patricia provided an account which helps to illustrate this theme. She continued teaching in the face of extreme pain in her back which rendered her unable to bend, and also pain resulting from appendicitis which was undiagnosed at the time. She spoke of how turning her head to speak to a student on the corridor could not be achieved without causing pain. During breaks, Patricia sought out a disused corridor to lie on the floor for relief from the pain. The traumatic impact of the physical illness is evident in her metaphoric use of the word *hell*. Giving up a well-paid job where she had earned praise for her teaching skills 'broke her heart'. She experienced suffering, grief, powerlessness, neglect, a lack of support, alienation and loss in her final stages of teaching:

> in between in the breaks in the class I used be lying on the corridor on a spare disused corridor trying to ease my back and I'd go back in and I'd be bending to look at their paper and then it would start and then you drop your pen ... and you wouldn't be able to bend to pick it up and you know walking down a corridor twisting to talk to the students would start off the pain you know it was just hell and actually, it was a few weeks before the appendix burst that I stopped you know but that killed me because it was a really good job I was getting paid 50 euros an hour.

Alice, who fell ill in her mid-twenties, terminated the relationship with her boyfriend because she had to rest and recuperate after work every day. She eventually lost her job after five years attempting to sustain employment:

> I think the worst thing was trying to continue life over those five years, in some sense, appearing to be somewhat normal, at that age, not knowing what was wrong, trying to appear normal to people, trying to kind of going to work, trying to focus on things, go home to bed having no life, it was a nightmare looking back on it, I think at that age you want to be doing things and I couldn't.

Orla was sixteen when she fell ill. She expressed a sense of loss of her youth and missing her debutantes' ball. She endured the stress resulting from trying to study and sit exams with permanent influenza-like symptoms. Orla also spoke of the strain of her perseverance during school and university in the face of undiagnosed and untreated debilitating illness amidst a feeling of desperation about the incomprehension surrounding her illness.

> I was so young when I got ill, I was 16, and it really affected my exams. Then when I went to university I was ok for the first year, but the second year I was knocked out completely ... I had to really work hard to catch up because I was in bed and sick nearly that whole year.

The above accounts mirror my own experience of a protracted struggle to remain in the workplace in the face of ill health: 'Every morning I woke up exhausted', I wrote in my narrative about working life in London, 'dragged myself to the bus stop ... devoid of any energy before even going into the office.' This sense of unending exertion prevailed throughout my twenties until I found a partial solution in my thirties:

> At thirty-three, I set up a business, with the understanding that I would work when I was able to, and stay at home and rest when I was unable to function.

In order to illuminate the theme featured here, I turned to Susan Wendell, a philosopher and professor emerita of feminist social theory at Simon Frazer University in British Columbia, Canada, who, in a similar fashion, endeavoured to stay in the workplace in the face of ill health. She has recalled how she had enjoyed superb health, fitness and an impressive academic career until she became ill with ME. She has never regained full health. After two years of being virtually bedridden she recovered sufficiently to return to work on a part time basis, spending the rest of the time lying down to recuperate her energy. This experience led her to develop courses in the university on the topic of women and disability, and to broaden her feminist research base to include disability and chronic illness.

Although Wendell is a scholar in the field of feminist philosophy, she has admitted that she could find little to give her comfort in feminist thought when her health failed her. In her book *The Rejected Body: Feminist Philosophical Reflections on Disability* (1996), she described how she felt side-lined when she became ill: 'Good feminists, like good women everywhere, are supposed to give 'til it hurts; everyone is supposed to feel exhausted and overworked, so why should I be the exception?'[7]

Wendell found support and inspiration, however, by reading about people's experiences of disability. She found in disability literature a deep awareness on the part of people with disabilities about how 'their cultures treat rejected aspects of bodily life.'[8] Referring to the lack of this awareness in feminist theory, she stated, 'feminist theory of the body was consequently both incomplete and skewed towards healthy, non-disabled experience.'[9] In order to fill this gap, Wendell set about undertaking theorising on disability, and on chronic illness as a disability.

Wendell has argued that disability is socially constructed, and is defined and determined by our culture and society. Human beings are damaged by factors such as the consequences of wars, violence, poor nourishment, environmental factors and child abuse. Wendell posited that disability is created by societies that possess 'an unacknowledged assumption that everyone is healthy, non-disabled, young but adult, shaped according to cultural ideals, and, often, male'.[10] Those who do not fit into this paradigm are deemed *other* and *disabled*. She argued that the world of the workplace has been structured as though no-one has to breast-feed a baby or look after a child. The common cold is acknowledged, she added, whereas no allowances are made for painful menstruation.

7    S. Wendell, *The Rejected Body: Feminist Philosophical Reflections on Disability*, 1st edn (New York: Routledge, 1996), 4.
8    Ibid., 5.
9    Ibid.
10   Ibid.

Psychoanalyst and philosopher Julia Kristeva has also argued that the workplace is often highly problematic for women and men alike, as evidenced by her patients in psychoanalysis:

> Contrary to the propaganda with which globalized technology assaults us, the global age that has followed the modern age is not one of the high performance, pleasure-led Man, bisexual master of his desires, their debacles, or both. The vulnerability that is revealed today on the couch is precisely that which is determined to deny the manic invasion of hyperproductivity, all-pervasive spectacle, and suicidal religious warfare.[11]

As a sufferer of ME, Susan Wendell is particularly sensitive to the *pace of life* as a contributing factor to illness. She has argued that the more the pace of life increases, the more people will become disabled, as 'the physical (and mental) limitations of those who cannot meet the new pace become conspicuous and disabling, even though the same limitations were inconspicuous and irrelevant to full participation in the slower based society'.[12]

Wendell has argued that what is considered 'normal' is defined by those who are able to work and are healthy, young and able-bodied. She emphasised that the worlds of the 'paradigm' healthy and the worlds of the sick and disabled have become split: 'The public world is the world of strength, the positive (valued) body, performance and production, the non-disabled, and young adults. Weakness, illness, rest, recovery, pain, death and the negative (devalued) body are private, generally hidden, and are often neglected'.[13] A consequence of the split is that the experience of disability and illness goes underground, 'because there is no socially acceptable way of expressing it and having the physical and psychological experience acknowledged'.[14] It is noteworthy that the Papal Encyclical *Laudato Si* (2015) has challenged 'rapidification' and its impact on human well-being.[15]

---

11    J. Kristeva, *Hatred and Forgiveness*, European Perspectives (New York: Columbia University Press, 2010), 42.

12    Wendell, *The Rejected Body*, 1996, 37.

13    Ibid., 40.

14    Ibid., 40.

15    <http://w2.vatican.va/content/francesco/en/encyclicals/documents/papa-francesco_20150524_enciclica-laudato-si.html>. Accessed 18 October 2015.

## Trauma as a Consequence of Not Being Believed by Doctors

Not being believed by members of the medical profession constituted a theme in eight of the interviews and had varying features. Some of the women who hadn't been believed by their GPs changed to new GPs who believed them, but they weren't able to find consultants who believed them (this is often necessary for social welfare, treatment and other matters). Some were believed by overseas doctors who use different tests but home doctors did not believe the overseas doctors' test results. One respondent, though believed now after many years of not being believed, encountered a medical professional who stated there was no such disease as ME, with which she had been diagnosed. Another respondent who hadn't been believed for five years and was then believed, later developed another contested illness which the medical profession doesn't validate. Some have a feeling of not being believed by social welfare examining doctors, and one had her benefits cut off as a result of an examination. The ninth respondent, Rachel, represented the minority voice. Rachel was happy that she was believed by her doctor and by her consultant, but was dismayed that her consultant instructed her to insert 'depression' on her application form for early retirement, because insurance company doctors did not consider fibromyalgia, her diagnosis, as valid justification for taking early retirement.

A classic incident was described by Mary Rose who has ME, which is also sometimes referred to as *post-viral syndrome*, and she also has multiple chemical sensitivity. Though believed by three consultants in the past, she spoke of the random nature of being believed and related how during an emergency hospital visit her sense of vulnerability was compounded by comments made by a non-empathic consultant, and resulted in feelings of not being believed:

> My speech was coming and going and I said to the consultant, 'I have post-viral syndrome' and the consultant said to me, 'what is this post-viral syndrome?' I thought, 'my God how to explain that when I can't even talk right'. I found it very hard to get through to them that I couldn't tolerate medication, they see you as medication-phobic whereas in fact you are medication-sensitive.

The following vignette illustrates respondents' experiences of not being believed by the medical profession:

Mary Rose reported that she is believed by her own doctor, but when she has to go to hospital, she experiences her condition being negated by some of the hospital doctors. She added that she was believed by her former three consultants, but they have now retired or have moved on. She feels discredited by the new consultant. She has a feeling of anxiety if she has to deal with new doctors, and a dread of a lack of empathy from doctors pervades any dealings with the medical world; she spoke of the 'random nature' of doctors who validate her illness. Sally explained that she is believed by her doctor but was not believed by a consultant. She also stated that she was told in a non-empathic manner by a health official that ME, her diagnosis, does not exist. Angela's story was not believed by local doctors from the age of sixteen to thirty-eight. She travelled to the USA and had her narrative taken seriously by an American doctor who suspected TB. She returned home and was then believed by her doctors who tested her positive for TB and treated her for it. Alice spoke of being ill for five years, misdiagnosed with anorexia nervosa, and committed to a psychiatric unit. A visiting doctor suspected a bowel problem. Subsequent tests verified this and surgery rectified the issue. Alice's present condition, however, severe multiple chemical sensitivity, is a contested illness that is not recognised by many doctors. She explained how this leads to her feeling unsafe dealing with people she doesn't know in the medical world in case she encounters disbelief.

Sharon was not believed by her family doctor. She visited the USA, where she was diagnosed with Lyme disease. She returned to Ireland and found a GP who believed her. Even with positive Lyme disease test results from the USA she was not believed by an Irish consultant. Finally she found an Irish consultant who believed her and affirmed her overseas results, and was then able to obtain treatment. Orla was disbelieved by doctors as all tests undertaken showed no disease from the age of sixteen until her early twenties. Finally, doctors insisted on more sophisticated testing. After these tests she was believed and diagnosed with ME.

Patricia was not believed by doctors because her tests results did not show up any disease. As a consequence, her disability allowance was terminated. She lodged an appeal and the next doctor believed her and insisted on her benefits being reinstated. Rachel's diagnosis is fibromyalgia, and she has had no problems being taken seriously by doctors. However, a consultant, supporting her in her application for early retirement, advised her to state that her diagnosis was 'depression', rather than 'fibromyalgia' in her application form for early retirement, so that her request would be taken seriously. Julia was told by her doctor that her experiences of electro-sensitivity were imagined. She changed to a different doctor who had worked in Germany and was familiar with the condition. Electromagnetic hypersensitivity is a contested illness which renders her feeling not believed by the wider medical community. She gains a feeling of validation in the knowledge that the condition has some validity in Sweden.

This synopsis illustrates how each of the nine participants experienced the disbelieving medical world, and reveal inconsistency surrounding being believed, or not believed, by doctors. The random nature of being believed and the impression of a lack of empathy on the part of the doctors is experienced as a source of anxiety. Some illnesses which were not believed to be physical by the medical profession in Ireland were believed to be physical in some other countries. It is evident that respondents are affected in practical ways by lack of belief from the medical profession, on whom they depend for sick certificates, treatment, and social welfare. These accounts clearly show that respondents are at a disadvantage because their illness is not believed to be physical, or is a contested illness.

The crucial nature of a validating medical diagnosis featured in my personal experience of illness. The relief I felt when a highly empathic medical professor in Germany tested me positive for Lyme disease was reflected in some of the narratives, in particular, the testimonies from Angela, Sharon and Julia.

An article in *Philosophy, Ethics and Humanities in Medicine* in 2008 by Johanna Shapiro, professor at the University of California's School of Medicine, helped to illuminate the lack of empathy felt by the women. She queried why many medical students start out with high levels of empathy for the patient, but may be observed to have this quality of empathy decrease over time. What she concluded about medical students is equally applicable to other human beings and to society:

Despite its pivotal role in medical practice, the impulse to 'draw closer,' to become engaged and connected with the suffering other, is far from automatic in human nature. In fact, we have an equal, if not stronger, and opposite impulse to draw back, detach, and separate from the contamination of illness. This impulse may well be related to fear of our own suffering and death, and likely contains an historically important element of self-preservation. If we did not draw back from contagious disease or physical threat, we might easily encourage our own extinction.[16]

The withdrawal of empathy may be linked to post traumatic stress disorder. I conducted a search for literature which would illuminate the traumatic effect disbelief may have on an individual who is not just chronically ill, but has the added burden to bear of an illness whose validity is contested. Judith Herman broadened the definition of 'post-traumatic stress disorder' (PTSD), which until her ground-breaking work had been defined in psychiatry as a condition that developed as a result of exposure to one traumatic event. Herman proposed a designation of 'complex trauma' to describe the kind of traumatic experience resulting from prolonged or multiple exposures to traumatic incidences.[17] The term 'complex trauma' is applicable to sufferers of chronic invisible illnesses who experience multiple exposures to traumatic events, while their nervous systems are vulnerable and sensitivity is heightened. This excerpt from my personal narrative points to complex trauma:

At thirty-nine, I became very ill and was unable to sustain working any longer. I was sick all the time, with flu-like symptoms, a chest infection that wouldn't go away, and weakness and lack of energy. Partly due to my condition we lost our biggest client, and I did not have the energy or the motivation to replace that amount of lost revenue.

Herman has isolated the three categories of symptoms of post-traumatic stress disorder, *hyperarousal, intrusion* and *constriction*. Research conducted in 2009 has found that these symptoms are experienced on a continuous

---

16    J. Shapiro, 'Walking a Mile in Their Patients' Shoes: Empathy and Othering in Medical Students' Education', *Philosophy, Ethics, and Humanities in Medicine*, 12 March 2008, <http://www.ncbi.nlm.nih.gov/pmc/articles/PMC2278157/>. Accessed 22 November 2012.

17    Herman, *Trauma and Recovery*, 119.

basis by sufferers of ME and fibromyalgia.[18] In the aftermath of a traumatic incident, Herman observed, the human system manifests a permanent state of alert, as if the threat or danger will return at any time. The body is in a state of *hyperarousal:* 'The traumatised person startles easily, reacts irritably to small provocations, and sleeps poorly'.[19] This cluster of symptoms is a familiar feature for many people with ME.

Herman also postulated that long after the danger has passed, traumatised people re-live the event as though it was occurring in the present. This category of symptoms comes under the heading of *intrusion.* There is a frozen and wordless quality to the way in which the traumatic moment breaks spontaneously into consciousness, as flashbacks or nightmares. For those living with chronic illnesses, these intrusive memories can be about the pain of how they worked hard, holding onto a job long after they were able to, only to feel rejected in the end.

The third category of symptoms of PTSD elucidated by Herman was that of *constriction,* which she described as an alteration of consciousness that a person experiences when powerless. This response can be likened to the 'freeze' state which is a self-defence mechanism popularly known as the 'rabbit in the headlights' effect. Also labelled 'dissociation', this state has resemblance to hypnotic trance, together with numbness symptoms. This constrictive state keeps traumatic memories out of normal consciousness. Herman emphasised that the constrictive symptoms applied 'not only to thought, memory and states of consciousness but also to the entire field of purposeful action and initiative'.[20]

She posited that because re-living a traumatic experience provokes emotional distress, traumatised people will go to great lengths to avoid a similar experience. This attempt to stay clear of potential threats 'further aggravates the post-traumatic syndrome, for the attempt to avoid re-living

---

18    A. Ben-Zvi, S. Vernon, and G. Broderick, 'Model-Based Therapeutic Correction of Hypothalamic-Pituitary-Adrenal Axis Dysfunction', *PLoS Comput Biol* 5, no. 1 (23 January 2009): 1–10, <https://doi.org/10.1371/journal.pcbi.1000273>.

19    Herman, *Trauma and Recovery*, 35.

20    Ibid., 46.

the trauma too often results in a narrowing of consciousness, a withdrawal from engagement with others, and an impoverished life'.[21]

## Not Being Believed by Other People as a Result of Not Being Believed by Doctors

The lack of diagnosis of a physical disease, or being diagnosed with a contested illness, by the medical profession had adverse consequences for eight of the interviewees in respect of their relationships with family and the wider community. The ninth, Rachel, did not experience disbelief by doctors and was also believed by her husband, her mother, her family, friends and her wider community.

The lack of diagnosis renders the disease 'invisible' to the medical eye because it does not show up in standard tests. It has a correlation of invisibility in society also because diagnosis provides a certain protection, rank and dignity for people who are vulnerable. The absence of diagnosis led to respondents feeling vulnerable to criticism from other people and to being at the receiving end of expectations of being healthier and more active. Added to that, when the person is able to go out, for example to the shops, they often look healthy by virtue of the fact that they are well enough to go out. But, respondents pointed out, one outing can necessitate days of rest and recuperation.

Although participants experienced debility and illness, they felt there was an expectation that they should be in good health because the medical profession could find no disease.

Respondents expressed emotional pain, shame, feelings of stigma, alienation, injustice, rejection, disconnection, frustration, lack of trust and isolation in relation to their families and associates as a result of the lack of a credible diagnosis and its corresponding validation.

21    Ibid., 42.

Sharon stated that her family don't understand why she was still sick after so many years: 'It's like they can't understand after nine years that if there is something wrong with you, surely the doctors would have cured it by now.' In a similar fashion, Orla experienced relationship problems in her family. She recalls family support 'falling away', and comments in the vein of: 'if the doctors can't find anything there mustn't be anything there, so it must be psychological'. Julia incurred family relationship breakdown; one of her sons doesn't believe her, nineteen years after onset of ongoing intolerance to electricity, mobile phones and masts.

Alice grieved loss of friendship when a certain close friend would not believe her chemical sensitivity was real: 'To this day she doesn't believe in it. If I had a broken leg, she would be the kindest person and everything would be done for me, but she would never accept the chemical sensitivity.'

Mary Rose believes that when people comment on how well she looks there is an embedded expectation that she should be able to do more than she is doing. She explained that she often looks flushed and people misconstrue her rosy complexion: 'People think it's a healthy glow but when I have the red glow it actually means that I am actually ready to physically keel over and people can tell me just how well I look and they ask me: "Oh, can you drive to the sea?" I wouldn't be able to go as a passenger most of the time ... it could be just a case that you would be struggling to stand upright.' Sally too expressed frustration about people judging her apparently healthy appearance when she is outdoors in public: 'People don't see you when you're not outside the door, how do they get the real picture of what life is like?' Angela remarked that it's difficult to explain this illness to herself, let alone others: 'You don't know what the hell is happening to you, and everybody else is doing a jig around you saying "what's wrong with you?" And you can't explain it to anybody, let alone yourself, and so there you are with like all your own questions and everybody else's questions, like "what the hell is wrong with you?"' Patricia feels the pain of judgement and negation from others during the nights when pain keeps her awake: 'You'd be bitter in the small hours of the night when you are up with the pain and you are thinking that they are all sleeping, these people who say "there is nothing wrong with you", and you are up night after night after night and sometimes you feel so angry that you feel like calling them in the night and saying "by the way I am just up at the moment because I have pain!"'

These accounts from eight of the participants portray the adverse consequences in family life and in society of not being believed by the medical
profession. The quotations poignantly illustrate the women's distress that
they are expected be able to do more, and to recover sooner. Disbelief by
others and trivialisation of their illnesses resulted in self-doubt, confusion,
alienation, bitterness, loss of support, and family discord. Although the
word 'stigma' was not used by the participants, stigmatisation is evident
here. These findings corroborate with a study in 2002 by Swedish researchers Åsbring and Närvänen of twenty-five women diagnosed with CFS or
Fibromyalgia. The focus here was on whether these illnesses are stigmatising.
Stigmatisation was found to be most acute when the women experienced
their condition being psychologised. Participants found the act of prescrib-
ing antidepressants to be 'violating'. They also experienced chronic fatigue
syndrome and fibromyalgia as stigmatising in relation to others questioning
their morality, feeling that their moral character was called into question
by those who challenged the legitimacy of their condition.

> Questioning occurred, for example, at work, where they felt accused of being 'work
> shy'. Most women also felt that providers questioned their credibility after tests
> revealed no pathological problems. They felt that providers regarded them as malin-
> gerers, with concocted non-existent or exaggerated problems.[22]

As a consequence of stigmatisation, the study reported that the women
developed strategies to avoid stigma such as withdrawing from social life,
and from care providers, sometimes avoiding contact with the medical
profession. Others tried to maintain a façade of a healthy and happy individual, only to collapse on the couch when they returned home.

Dismissive attitudes from family members and others may be echoed
in an intrapsychic nature by the voices of an 'inner critic', which, identified with the voice of the doctor, mete out devastating judgements. As my
narrative illustrates, harsh opinions emanated from my inner critic about
my difficulty coping with life in the workplace:

---

22   Pia Asbring and Anna-Liisa Närvänen, 'Women's Experiences of Stigma in Relation
     to Chronic Fatigue Syndrome and Fibromyalgia', *Qualitative Health Research* 12,
     no. 2 (February 2002): 148–60, <https://doi.org/10.1177/104973230201200202>.

My interpretation of this at the time was that I needed to 'get a grip'. I thought I was lazy and lethargic. I gave up coffee, tried the gym, Pilates and swimming, pushing myself hard to become energetic. None of those approaches were beneficial.

The investigations of Michel Foucault (1926–1984), a French philosopher who theorised on normativity and deliberated on the notion of medicine as a tool of subtle social control, may help us to understand the theme being treated here.[23] Foucault suggested that modern individuals are controlled by standards of normality which are laid down by professions which assess and diagnose people, such as medicine, psychology and psychiatry. His metaphoric 'regard médical' or 'clinical gaze', represented the authority of medicine to read and diagnose the human body and the way in which other people adopt such diagnoses and assessments as 'truth'. This leads to individuals internalising the diagnoses and becoming collaborating agents in labelling what is 'normal'. His publication, *Naissance de la Clinique: une Archéologie du Regard Médical* [*The Birth of the Clinic: An Archaeology of Medical Perception*] first published in 1963, traced the history of medicine and the power invested by people in the medical profession.[24]

## Hurtful Comments Made by Members of the Medical Profession

The following account illustrates the theme of negative comments or attitudes on the part of the medical profession. Eight respondents conveyed a sense of being put down, of neglect, shock, offense, stigmatisation, alienation, despair, separation, abandonment, anxiety, shame and disbelief at the way they had been treated. While the ninth, Rachel, who was believed,

23  M. Foucault, *The Order of Things: An Archaeology of the Human Sciences*, 1st edn (New York: Vintage, 1994).

24  M. Foucault, *Naissance de la Clinique*, PUF edition (Paris: Presses Universitaires de France, 2000).

did not convey an overall feeling of being dismissed, she experienced being unsettled by some words from her consultant:

> He said, 'You have fibromyalgia ... it is typical of women, IMP – Intense Meticulous and Perfectionist' and he went on, 'I want you to read a book if you agree with the contents of the book (penned by the same doctor), come back in three weeks if you don't, don't bother coming back at all.'

Sally remembers a time when she still had faith in the medical profession, even when she felt that her reality was being denied by doctors: 'I lost a lot of control over a lot of bodily functions quite suddenly and they said "Oh there is nothing wrong with you". At that point I trusted the medical profession still. I thought, "Well, maybe they are right, maybe I just need a break or something", so I rested and I did all sorts of positive things but I only became more and more ill.'

Angela, years after the event, still displayed a sense of shock that a consultant had belittled her experience: '"Ah you'll be all right", an endocrinologist said to me, "you will be grand; just go and find yourself a husband and get a few children for yourself", and at this point like my menstruation had even stopped.' Sharon recalled a similar experience with a consultant: 'I was sent to a specialist who charged me €180 and more or less suggested that I got a few hobbies to get me out of the house more.'

Alice, who was diagnosed with anorexia nervosa but who was later found to have volvulus, commonly referred to as a 'twisted bowel', recounted a conversation her psychiatrist had with her father: 'He just told my father that there was nothing wrong with me, I needed a good kick up the backside, but I couldn't eat. They told me I had anorexia.' Patricia described a scene where she felt humiliated whilst being examined by a male doctor representing the social welfare department in a consultation to determine whether or not she was entitled to benefits: 'He said to me "I want you to bend" so when I went to bend I automatically put my hand on the chair, because that's one of my problems is bending, I can bend if I bend very carefully, but I can't bend too far, I must use support. He said: "Take your hand off the back of the chair." So, I said to him, "It's kind of less likely the pain will start". He said, "Just bend." I didn't know whether he wanted me to bend to the point of the pain or to bend and start the pain so I started asking him about it. He said, "It's not very complicated," he said, "I mean if you like I'll look away." Julia, the retired nurse who suffers from severe electro-sensitivity, expressed incredulity that her family doctor didn't believe her: 'He said "I am an orthodox doctor". "Well", I said, "I was an orthodox nurse until this hit me"'.

These ways in which the women were subjected to disrespectful remarks by doctors clearly show how, because of the 'invisibility' of their illnesses, they felt shamed, disempowered and stigmatised. It is evident that they felt violated and degraded by the trivialisation of their illness and by being told by male doctors to find a husband, have children, to take up hobbies and to rest and do positive things. A sense of the violation of the dignity of the women is tangible in a remark concerning an illness being typical of a female who was intense, meticulous, and perfectionist, while another was told she needed a kick in the backside.

This theme of hurtful comments on the part of the medical profession highlights a distinctly sexist attitude towards the women. In a similar fashion, I have experienced feelings of negation by the medical profession. The following excerpts from letters from a consultant to my GP were particularly disconcerting:

> Both Dr Smith (the consultant) and myself feel that there is most likely a super-centorial aspect to this however we are anxious to exclude an organic cause before labelling her with this.[25]

I have been unable to find a definition of the word 'supercentorial' in any dictionary on the internet; however, a word with a slightly different spelling 'supracentorial' denotes an anatomical region of the brain. In any case, the context in which the word is used infers that the illness was psychological in nature and that other diseases, for which they could find an organic cause, are not. A subsequent letter from the same consultant added weight to this notion:

> Again I feel it is most likely that this lady's symptoms are psychological in nature ... I have asked her to discuss with you in the coming months the possibility of starting

25    Extract from a letter to my GP, July 2004.

her on another course of anti-depressant medications in the hope that this might improve her symptoms. She has taken anti-depressants in the past without any definite improvement in her energy levels though at this point it is probably worth trying a further course ... for two or three months.[26]

A clinical psychologist from Seattle, Maria Root, proposed a model of *insidious trauma* to theorise on the effects of forms of oppression that are not overtly violent or physically threatening, but which do violence to the soul or spirit.[27] Her work emerged out of the field of ethnic minority psychology and theorises that many marginalised people suffer hurtful comments and insults in everyday life which build up and amount to trauma for those populations. Root argues that this type of trauma may be a feature in instances of chronic illness, 'Insidious trauma may also occur with the experience of significantly declining health, progressive debilitating illness, or markedly decreased ability to function independently (e.g. in AIDS, diabetes, multiple sclerosis, some cancers).'[28] Comments on how well she looked led to the publication of a popular 2005 self-help book called *You Don't Look Sick: Living Well with Invisible Chronic Illness*, penned by Joy Selak, who has an invisible illness.[29]

Maria Root's conceptualisation of *insidious* trauma offers a framework for the way in which marginalisation and stigmatisation traumatise the wounded person in so many facets of her life. The sufferer of chronic illness even feels excluded listening to the radio; the programmes are broadcast from the studios of the kingdom of the well, to use a metaphor from an author who suffered from cancer, Susan Sontag: 'Everyone who is born holds dual citizenship, in the kingdom of the well and in the kingdom of the sick.'[30]

---

26   Extract from a letter to my GP, August 2004.
27   M. Root, 'Reconstructing the Impact of Trauma on Personality', in *Personality and Psychopathology: Feminist Reappraisals*, eds L. Brown and Mary Ballou Ballou, reprint edn (New York: The Guilford Press, 1994), 229.
28   Ibid., 241.
29   J. Selak, *You Don't Look Sick!: Living Well with Invisible Chronic Illness* (New York: Haworth Medical Press, 2005).
30   S. Sontag, *Illness as Metaphor* (New York: Vintage Books, 1979), 3.

## Trauma of Losses through Illness

All nine interviewees spoke of the loss of career and life opportunities. Six of the respondents spoke about the difficulty around having a relationship with a partner because of their health. Sharon contributed one explanation: 'I'm not really able to sustain a relationship because there's very few men who could understand what it is to not have any energy.' Julia is unable to live with her husband because of the radiation in the family home from masts and electricity. The theme of difficulty having a relationship with a partner due to illness did not arise in the other three narratives.

A central loss to all nine was that of career opportunities. Mary Rose, a former teacher, now in her early fifties, reminisced about how she used to love to socialise: 'I loved plays and going out to different societies and I loved to travel. I even lost my sense of self for a long time because your sense of self image is so bound up with what your role is in life, and your job.' Sally misses the fulfilment she enjoyed working with boys with mental health issues, describing a sense of a job unfinished: 'The year that I got ill I had started working in a group home with kids with difficulties. I did art with them and I started making puppets with them. Unfortunately I still, I mean it's 15 years ago and I still feel I need to finish it with them. These guys are probably now married and having kids but I still feel that it was broken.' Patricia spoke of the self-esteem generated by her work as a teacher: 'It broke my heart I had to give that up, but that was great for my confidence because the woman there told me that I was the best teacher, you know. That was great to hear that and I kind of cling on to that.' Similarly Rachel described giving up work as the lowest point: 'I can see now with the wisdom of hindsight the sense of myself was completely bound in with being a teacher, the scholarship girl, that's human – we have to develop an image to live, but I found that loss excruciating.' Julia's sense of loss is tightly bound up with her years of dedication to the medical profession as a nurse, a job she loved. Her major hurt was that a profession to which she devoted her life didn't give her the credence she required of them when she became ill with severe electromagnetic sensitivity. This loss of the support of the medical profession was experienced by Julia as a death: 'I said to myself "if this is what it's like to be dead I am dead". And I didn't know where I was going, just I was that I was dead really to what I knew.'

Angela acutely felt a loss of a healthy transformation into womanhood: 'It was totally traumatic to be transitioning into womanhood and transitioning into menstruation, and at the same time manifesting like a horrible illness, a horrible illness, because it took me 20 years to get a diagnosis, it took all of my 20s, and half of my 30s, before I finally got someone to figure out what was wrong with me.' Alice described wistfully the normal things of youth that were taken from her: 'I was just beginning to go out and enjoy life, and I had a nice boyfriend at the time, and I was going off on holidays ... and it was before I went to Greece that I got sick but I went, and I just was very sick after and it was when I came home I just didn't know what was wrong, I had lost weight and I couldn't swallow, I couldn't eat, I was losing weight. I spent the next five years looking for an answer to that. That was the worst part of my life.' In a similar vein, Orla mourns the loss of a healthy adolescence: 'When I see the life that some teenagers have now, how they are going out, my nieces are involved in really interesting projects ... I couldn't really do any of that, I was too sick, and that's a loss.'

Sharon tries hard to re-build a relationship with her daughters. She wept openly when she revealed that her biggest loss was relationship with them: 'When they were 16 and 17 and they needed me, I wasn't able to be there for them, because I was sick. That's my biggest loss is the loss of being able to be a mother. I spent any money I had on my treatment. I didn't send them to college; all of my savings went on my treatment so my girls basically left school early. I don't really feel that I am even their mother now. When they talk about home, home isn't here – home is their aunt's house.'

This narrative illustrates the vast losses endured by each of the participants as a result of their illnesses. It is clear that illness has cost them extensive losses in their careers and in their personal lives. There is vivid sense of ongoing years of a blank canvas, mourning for lost teenage years, lost chances of being in a relationship, loss of capability to mother teenage daughters, loss of trust, unfinished business, and loss of a sense of self which was bound to their careers.

My own sense of loss in illness mirrors the experiences recounted above. Relocating from London to rural Ireland, being unemployed due to illness, appear in the narrative in stark contrast to a television career in London: 'I had no friends my own age, or with similar interests, in the area. I felt like a fish out of water, conspicuous, living alone in a strange village.'

## Enduring Quotidien Trauma

Trauma associated with everyday living with chronic illness permeated eight of the nine narratives. The ninth spoke of relief due to medication and experienced family support. The harrowing nature of the daily experience of illness was emphasised by Angela who avowed, 'when you have had too many downtimes in your life you doubt your sanity.'

A constant feature in Sally's life is the anxiety that accompanies a poor and fluctuating level of health which requires hospitalisation from time to time. She also has a fear of falling, a fear of attitudes of some of the medical profession, and the strain of not having access to the treatments she would like due to poverty or lack of availability. She feels she does not get the help she needs and is hoping to go overseas for help if she can get financial support. 'With ME you just have to scramble to get people to understand, to get the help.' Though she has had treatment for TB and a hip replacement, Angela struggles with fatigue, nausea, weakness and fluctuating health. 'I feel like it's a constant dance with health ... I feel like I am sort of on some kind of knife edge all the time.' She has visited clinics in Europe for help but struggles to implement their programme due to lack of money. She feels the strain of the ongoing expectations and comments from people about her illness. Alice's health stresses involve not being capable of concentrating on the telephone for more than 30 minutes. She showed anguish when talking about when she was committed to a psychiatric hospital in her twenties, and, in the aftermath of our interview, she experienced flashbacks. 'I am sick since I was 24, but I am now 65 so I don't know anything else, I have always not been able to do things, not be able to do this, not been able to do that, always tired, always trying to pace myself.' Paucity of income makes it difficult to avail of organically grown foods and holistic treatments, which would help her. On any outing, she remains alert for chemical toxins such as paint, plug-in air fresheners, and people wearing perfume and after-shave lotion. An encounter with pollutants leads to severe muscle spasms. The consequences of an encounter with chemicals, for example in shops, clinics or hospitals might not appear for days so she experiences the stress of not knowing how she will be at any time. The isolating effect is further compounded by the shame that comes from the lack of standing of chemical sensitivity as an illness.

Daily stresses for Sharon include 'brain fog' symptoms, memory loss, low energy, weakness and nausea. She described enduring 'constant unremitting fatigue and terrible blinding headaches.' Coping with the bureaucracy involved in applying for medical benefits, form-filling followed by a lengthy appeal process, and difficulty getting a consultant to support her application, were examples she gave of the stress and sense of abandonment she felt in daily life. She spoke also of the embarrassment of being means-tested for her medical card by a male official with whom she had been acquainted in her business life. She feels isolated and cannot stay on the phone for long periods. She experiences stress when family members come to stay because she doesn't have energy for the company, but mourns their loss when they are absent. She spoke too of the financial strain that illness brings and its consequences for her family. Orla now works one day a week but feels she has lost out on promotions and the respect that her peers have enjoyed.

Patricia moved to the countryside because of debilitating allergies. She is unable to spend much time on the phone due to fatigue, and she feels isolated. She struggles with finance. Her poor health prevents her from visiting family. She is the object of prejudice from family members. Her insomnia is another feature of chronic trauma, the pain keeps waking her up, 'I'll fall [asleep], and I'll wake up ... My friend says to me, "In Guantanamo that's what they used to torture people, they keep waking them up!"' Rachel talked about ongoing excruciating pain up until not long before the research encounter, and was finding relief at the time of the interview as a result of new medication. Julia's pain due to electromagnetic sensitivity is a persistent stressor. Stress is caused by the fluctuating nature of the strength of radiation emissions. In addition, electric fences are switched on and off by nearby farmers, causing pain. She estimates that she has moved fifty times since her illness began and suffers stress on a daily basis not knowing where she will be able to spend the night. She explained one experience, 'I shifted my bed from the bedroom; I shifted it all around the bedroom ... the other two bedrooms. I went down to the sitting room and my husband came down one morning, and I was in under the kitchen table. He asked, "what are you doing here?" I said, "I have been pushing this thing [sun lounger bed] around all night", because the electricity was coming in under the ground. And in the end, I went off into the doctor again and I said to him, "Look, give me something." He said "I can't treat you, what you have is bizarre."'

Mary Rose suffers unpredictable bouts of severe illness that lead to hospitalisation, which causes anxiety partly because she has to wear a mask in the hospital to protect her from inhaling chemicals; she also fears not being believed, and the stigma of looking different as a result of wearing the mask. She related her daily anxiety, 'The trauma of all the physical frightening symptoms, the trauma of feeling kind of powerless, the trauma of feeling things could never get better, the trauma of other people not understanding you at times, the trauma of dealing with the medical system, the trauma of dealing with the insurance system when I needed my income, and being sent for medicals to prove I was sick.'

This account illustrates how the body is under a constant state of alertness due to the unpredictability of the illnesses. The illnesses bring fears: fear of falling, fear of hospitalisation, fear of medical examinations for social welfare or insurance purposes, and fear of an encounter with chemicals. In addition, isolation, poverty, and the bureaucracy of dealing with the social welfare system causes overwhelming stress when the body is unwell.

The sense of pervasive trauma evident in these accounts of contested illnesses echoes the perpetual nature of the trauma which suffuses my personal narrative and which may be detected in the following excerpt:

> I wondered is this it? Is this my life? The winters were hard, hard on the chest. Hard on the ego as I seemed to be drifting and have no status.

Yet it is the challenge presented by harsh experiences of perpetual daily trauma and marginalisation, as experienced by these women, which may become a gateway to spiritual awakening. Contemporary philosopher Ken Wilber, who has been open about his own chronic illness and suffering, conceived of suffering as a grace:

> For suffering smashes to pieces the complacency of our normal fictions about reality, and forces us to become alive in a special sense – to see carefully, to feel deeply, to touch ourselves and our worlds in ways we have heretofore avoided. It has been said, and I truly think, that suffering is the first grace. In a special sense, suffering is almost a time of rejoicing, for it marks the birth of creative insight.[31]

Texas-based clinical psychologist, Robert Grant, has worked as a trauma consultant in several disaster zones around the world and trains doctors, nurses, psychotherapists, and members of the police force who care for trauma victims. Having a background in clinical and organisational psychology, Grant considers trauma to be a unique catalyst for spiritual awakening in our world today. In his book *The Way of the Wound: A Spirituality of Growth and Transformation* (1999), Grant's focus is on the opportunity trauma provides for spiritual awakening. In contrast to many other trauma theorists, he has acknowledged illness as a source of trauma.[32] His approach to trauma is psycho-spiritual. He proposes that trauma may provide an opportunity for the ego to accept that it must become a servant of, instead of being a master of, the psyche:

> In the current Zeitgeist (spirit of the times) the ego is the only reality most victims have ever known. Normally it takes the gut-wrenching pain of trauma to expose the ego's limitations.[33]

---

31   K. Wilber, *No Boundary: Eastern and Western Approaches to Personal Growth* (Boston, MA: Shambhala, 2001), 76.

32   R. Grant, *The Way of the Wound: A Spirituality of Trauma and Transformation* (Burlingame, CA: self-published, 1999), 48.

33   Ibid., 100.

He saw trauma as a call to transformation, to align with a higher reality, that of the Spirit. The next section explores the myriad ways in which spiritual awakening, personal growth and transformation featured as outcomes of the trauma of chronic invisible illness for the women who participated in the study.

# CHAPTER 4

# The Discourses of Spiritual Awakening

> Our way of life has become meditative because we can't put up with the
> hurly burly, it makes us more receptive to spirit.
>
> — MARY ROSE

The term *spiritual awakening* identifies an opening in the awareness of the
human person to a 'higher' or 'deeper' dimension of human experience
which may be characterised by a stronger contact with inwardness and transcendence. Evelyn Underhill (1875–1941), a pioneer in the academic study
of mysticism, and the first woman lecturer at Oxford University, dedicated
a chapter to its elucidation in her foundational book *Mysticism: the Nature
and Development of Spiritual Consciousness*[1] which was first published in
1911. Underhill delineated five stages in spiritual development, the first of
which was the *awakening of the self to consciousness of Divine reality*. The
other four stages of the mystical path in her framework comprised of *purgation, illumination, mystic death* or *dark night of the soul* and, finally, *union
with the Divine*. But only the first stage is of concern to this discussion.

Underhill described the stage of awakening as a disturbance in the
equilibrium of the self, which results in the shifting of the field of consciousness from lower to higher levels, with a consequent removal of the
centre of interest from the subject to an object now brought into view:
the necessary beginning of any process of transcendence.[2] She expressed
reservations about any classification or mapping of the terrain of the soul,

---

1   E. Underhill, *Mysticism: The Nature and Development of Spiritual Consciousness.*
    (Oxford: One World, 1993).
2   Ibid., 176.

emphasising that: 'The creative impulse in the world, so far as we are aware of it, appears upon ultimate analysis to be free and original, not bound and mechanical'.[3] She insisted that her characterisations would be construed as, 'only answering loosely and generally to experiences which seldom present themselves in so rigid and unmixed a form'.[4]

Underhill went to great lengths to ensure that awakening would not be identified with religious conversion, and to emphasise that the results of awakening belonged to 'a higher order of reality'.[5] The awakening process implied not just the initial phenomenon but also entailed, 'the consequent remaking of the field of consciousness, an alteration in the self's attitude to the world'.[6]

American psychiatrist, Gerald May (1940–2005), authored a number of scholarly works on psycho-spiritual theory,[7] but it was in his popular book, *The Awakened Heart*, first published in 1991, that he devoted space to the awakening phase. Describing the diverse nature of awakenings, May stated: 'Some awakenings come in flashes, but more often we awaken in stages, as if emerging from a dream'.[8]

For the purposes of this research topic, the term *spiritual awakening* indicates the initial phenomenon of becoming aware of a spiritual dimension to existence, in conjunction with the ongoing sustaining of the state of being 'awakened' and of experiencing the integration of the insights gifted by that state. It encompasses the awakening, the staying awake and the state of wakefulness. In his introduction to mindfulness, *Mindfulness for Beginners: Reclaiming the Present Moment – and Your Life* (2011), Jon Kabat-Zinn, Emeritus Professor of Medicine at the University of Massachusetts Medical School, who promoted *mindfulness* in the West,

---

3    E. Underhill, *Mysticism* (Oxford: One World, 1993), 167.
4    Ibid., 168.
5    Ibid., 176.
6    Ibid., 177.
7    G. May, *Will and Spirit: A Contemplative Psychology*, reprint edn (San Francisco, CA; London: HarperOne, 1987); G. May, *Care of Mind/Care of Spirit: A Psychiatrist Explores Spiritual Direction*, Reprint edition (San Francisco, CA: HarperOne, 1992).
8    G. May, *The Awakened Heart*, reprint edn (San Francisco, CA: HarperOne, 1993), 50.

used the expression *wakefulness* to represent the condition of one who is in a constant state of being awakened.[9] In this study, spiritual awakening connotes not just the initial awakening phenomenon but the ongoing journey of ever unfolding wakefulness, which in turn implies a continuous engagement on deeper levels with the five stages charted by Underhill.

## An Emerging Discourse

There are many possible meanings of the word 'spirituality' as it relates to spiritual awakening. The definition used in this study borrows from one formulated by Christopher Cook, Professor of Spirituality, Theology and Health at Durham University:

> a distinctive, potentially creative and universal dimension of human experience arising both within inner subjective awareness of individuals and within communities, social groups, and traditions. It may be experienced as relationship with that which is intimately 'inner', immanent and personal, within the self and others, and/or as relationship with that which is wholly 'other', transcendent and beyond the self. It is experienced as being of fundamental or ultimate importance and is thus concerned with matters of meaning and purpose in life, truth and values.[10]

Cook admitted that this definition was somewhat lengthy and lacked precision;[11] nevertheless it has the advantages that it can be applied to people of all faiths or of no faith and recognises the universal dimension of spirituality. It does not identify spirituality with religion. Whilst acknowledging that the two subjects are related and overlap in various ways, Cook insisted that they also need to be distinguished from each other.

---

9   J. Kabat-Zinn, *Mindfulness for Beginners: Reclaiming the Present Moment – and Your Life*, 1st edn (Boulder, CO: Sounds True, 2011), 22.

10   C. Cook, 'Addiction and Spirituality', *Addiction* 99, no. 5 (May 2004): 593–51.

11   C. Cook, 'How Spirituality Is Relevant to Mental Healthcare and Ethical Concerns', 2013, <http://www.rcpsych.ac.uk>. Accessed 7 October 2014.

Spiritual awakening is not *sui generis* and so in a cognate manner the human maturation process can be conceptualised as a series of awakenings to higher or deeper states of consciousness. American psychologist Abraham Maslow (1908–1970) regarded the human being as having a hierarchy of needs which drive the development process.[12] When one need is fulfilled, a higher need presents itself to which the person is awakened. Moving from basic needs upwards, Maslow categorised those needs as pertaining to: physiological, safety, belongingness and love, esteem, self-actualisation and self-transcendence needs. He theorised that human motivations move through these layers and that when the human person's more basic physiological needs are satisfied, boredom can set in. When there is a sense of safety, belonging, love and esteem, a sense of ennui can ensue.

It is also worth considering here the work of Viktor Frankl (1905–1997), a psychiatrist who survived the Auschwitz concentration camp and who went on to become Professor of Neurology and Psychiatry at Vienna Medical School. Frankl labelled the phenomenon of ennui and meaninglessness the *existential vacuum*. He argued against this ennui and meaningless being equated to a mental disorder, but he suggested that it could be viewed instead as an attempt by the person's psyche to awaken to another higher or deeper state of consciousness: 'The existential vacuum', he wrote, 'is no neurosis; or, if it is a neurosis at all, it is a sociogenic neurosis, or even an iatrogenic neurosis – that is to say, a neurosis which is caused by the doctor who pretends to cure it'.[13]

Similarly, contemporary scholarly work in transpersonal theory and psycho-spiritual/contemplative psychology such as that of Ken Wilber, Stanislav Grof, Christina Grof, Roberto Assagioli, Thomas Merton, Gerald May, Carol Christ, Rosemarie Anderson, and Cynthia Bourgeault affirms this attempt by the psyche to awaken to a spiritual dimension of human existence. Awakening and staying awake to this level provides a level of functioning that enables the individual to operate from transpersonal

12    A. Maslow, 'A Theory of Human Motivation', *Psychological Review* 50, no. 4 (1943): 370–96, <https://doi.org/10.1037/h0054346>.

13    V. Frankl, *The Will to Meaning: Foundations and Applications of Logotherapy*, Rei Exp edn (New York: Plume, 1988), 88.

values such as love of humankind, justice, authenticity, deeper creativity, compassion, forgiveness, and appreciation of beauty and of the ecosystem. Conversely a denial of the existence of the transpersonal dimension, or a lack of awakening to it, can leave the individual believing that there is something wrong with her when she suffers this meaninglessness, depression and boredom, something she perceives that needs to be cured by medicine. Indeed, Western society as a whole tends to suffer from a denial of the transpersonal dimension.

Maria Harris (1932–2005) was a pioneer in religious education who is credited with re-shaping how religion is taught. She was a prolific author who left a legacy of scholarly books and articles in which she had developed her theories on religious education, women's spirituality, feminism and other topics. For the purposes of this research, however, I have chosen to focus on a popular self-help book she penned on women's spiritual development – *Dance of the Spirit: The Seven Steps of Women's Spirituality* – because of its attention to the awakening phase. In addition, at the time of publication in 1989, Harris's seven-step model, set out in this book, and her contention that women's spiritual development differed to that of men, was innovative and ground-breaking.[14]

## Maria Harris on Spiritual Awakening

Maria Harris counted awakening as the first step into an intentional spiritual life and also as an ongoing process which, once the awakening has happened, exists in a sustained manner.[15]

According to Harris, spiritual awakening is a movement toward transformation in the inner life of a woman. In the prologue to her book *The Dance of the Spirit: The Seven Stages of Women's Spirituality*, Harris discussed

14  M. Harris, *Dance of the Spirit: The Seven Stages of Women's Spirituality*, reprint edn (New York: Bantam, 1991).
15  Ibid., 30.

how during the previous twenty years she had witnessed 'a quiet revolution. That revolution is the rebirth of a genuine women's spirituality, which takes seriously the major issues in women's lives.'[16] The major issues which she discussed include: brokenness, connection, power, love, work and death. She discussed the essence of the seven steps of the spiritual dance, providing exercises and meditations for each stage.

Harris envisioned the spiritual journey of a woman as a dance rather than a linear movement. The seven steps of this dance, together with a brief synopsis of the meaning of each step, were summarised as follows:

1. Awakening: This first movement is concerned with awakening to feelings and the inner life. In this step, layers of demand, resistance and rigidity that have been built up over the years become brittle and begin to dissolve.
2. Dis-Covering: This involves a new self-accepting awareness of one's unique self.
3. Creating: This step relates to the discovery and development of one's unique creative capacity.
4. Dwelling: This central step of the dance concerns finding and resting in a sacred dwelling-place within, and practising awareness of the present moment.
5. Nourishing: Here, a commitment is made to spiritual disciplines such as prayer and meditation, so as to enhance capacities for attentiveness and awareness.
6. Traditioning: This movement embraces the passing on to others of the gift of spirituality, by actions such as mentoring.
7. Transforming: This final step involves the birth of a renewed sense of self.

After the seventh step, the dance begins again with the first step as the woman once again experiences awakening to a deeper level of awareness.

Maria Harris traced occurrences of the metaphor of awakening in Western spirituality to the Hebrew Bible and the New Testament. She

16    Ibid., xi.

asserted that the Hebrew Bible is not only an appeal to waken to the inner life but also to others who are in need. Harris considered the psalms as a call to awaken to a loving and attentive Divine listener who is available to assist in the journey being undertaken. Harris also highlighted the metaphors in the New Testament which pertained to awakening such as Paul's exhortation to the Romans, 'You know what hour it is, how it is full time now for you to wake from sleep. The night is far gone, the day is at hand' (Rom. 13:11–12).

Turning her gaze East, Harris observed awakening as a core theme especially in Zen Buddhism where awakening is a kind of knowing that is not of the territory of facts and data. In Zen, nature is imbued with a sacred presence: 'Everything is assumed capable of holding the sacred' and thus a robin or a tree can become spiritual companions.[17] This teaching has been underscored by renowned Vietnamese Zen Buddhist Thích Nhất Hạnh in a reminder to his followers that the vision of a practising Buddhist must include respect for every aspect of the ecosystem, 'trees, birds, violet bamboos, and yellow chrysanthemums are all preaching the same dharma that Shakyamuni taught 2,500 years ago.'[18]

Maria Harris appreciated Zen wisdom which teaches that a person can become more herself by allowing an object in nature to become more itself. She encouraged her students to adopt a practice of playing with nature by chanting by a lake, 'I see the lake, the lake sees me.' This is a type of Zen *koan* or philosophical riddle designed to enable the subject to awaken to a spiritual level of consciousness.[19] A teaching of Isan Reiyū (771–853), a Zen master of the Igyō school of Zen in China, who asked his pupil Kyōgen one day to go away and find an answer to the question, 'what is your essential face before your father and mother were born?', highlights the enigmatic character of *koans*.[20]

---

17  Ibid., 7.
18  Thích Nhất Hạnh, *For a Future to Be Possible: Buddhist Ethics for Everyday Life*, revised edn (Berkeley, CA: Parallax Press, 2007), 95.
19  Harris, *Dance of the Spirit*, 7.
20  K. Yamada and R. Habito, *The Gateless Gate: The Classic Book of Zen Koans* (Boston, MA: Wisdom Publications, 2004), 32.

## The Influence of Meister Eckhart

Harris's approach was influenced by Meister Eckhart (1260–1328), the Dominican theologian and mystic from Cologne. She considered his teaching on the spiritual life as essentially a call to awakening. Significantly, Eckhart had himself been profoundly affected by the writings of the Beguine women mystics.

Maria Harris did not extensively elaborate on the significance of Meister Eckhart regarding women's spiritual awakening. However, her incipient ideas are in line with those developed by Bernard McGinn, theologian and scholar on Meister Eckhart, who is affiliated with the University of Chicago. It will be worth elaborating on McGinn's scholarship on Eckhart here for the purpose of the illumination of Harris's discourse on women's spiritual life.

Bernard McGinn has investigated themes common to the writings of Eckhart and the women mystics Marguerite Porete, Hadewijch of Brabant and Mechthild of Magdeburg. A Dominican and spiritual director, Eckhart had been given theological control over the spiritual lives of Beguines and other nuns and laywomen but, instead of dominating their thinking, he incorporated their wisdom into his teaching and in this way respected the rising spiritual aspirations they embodied. Their theology has been termed *vernacular* because of its articulation in the local languages of its practitioners. This vernacular theological expression, the origins of which McGinn has traced to the twelfth century, had become 'a flood' by the thirteenth.[21] Its writings bore witness to the creation of a theological discourse accessible to the laity and to women, in particular women of the poorer classes, who were deprived of schooling in Latin. Writing in the vernacular was revolutionary at the time and enabled the women mystics to express the inner dimensions of their spiritual awakening: 'the explosion of religious writing in the vernacular was not just a case of simple translation, but was

---

21    B. McGinn, *Meister Eckhart and the Beguine Mystics: Hadewijch of Brabant, Mechthild of Magdeburg, and Marguerite Porete* (New York: The Continuum Publishing Company, 2001), 8.

a complex and still inadequately studied creation of new theological and linguistic possibilities.'[22] According to McGinn, it was in this vernacular tradition that, 'women, for the first time in the history of Christianity, took on an important, perhaps even a preponderant role'.[23]

Bernard McGinn maintains that Meister Eckhart was predisposed to the writing of women mystics such as Marguerite Porete (1250–1310), a Beguine mystic whom he had never met and who had been publicly burned to death as a heretic.[24] The Beguines were part of a lay Christian spiritual movement in northern Europe chiefly between the thirteenth and sixteenth centuries who lived in semi-monastic communities. Membership was made up of women who lived in spiritual companionship but who didn't take some of the vows associated with religious life. Indeed, many couldn't afford the dowry necessary to become a nun. Free from Church authorities, Beguines usually committed to a life of celibacy, prayer, contemplation and charitable works. The movement was, however, condemned in 1311 by Pope John XXII. The Beguine movement, created by and for lay women, which produced some of the most challenging religious texts of the middle ages, has garnered significant attention in recent years. In *Cities of Ladies: Beguine Communities in the Medieval Low Countries, 1200–1565*, published in 2001, Walter Simons, history professor at Dartmouth University, has assembled much of the research that had been generated over the previous fifty years.[25] In addition, Saskia Murk-Jansen, a Cambridge lecturer in medieval women's mysticism, has chronicled the development of the movement, highlighting its influence and the way in which it was repressed by Church authorities.[26]

---

22  Ibid., 7.
23  Ibid., 6.
24  Ibid., 2.
25  W. Simons, *Cities of Ladies: Beguine Communities in the Medieval Low Countries, 1200–1565*, Middle Ages Series (Philadelphia: University of Pennsylvania Press, 2001).
26  S. Murk-Jansen, *Brides in the Desert: The Spirituality of the Beguines*, Traditions of Christian Spirituality (Maryknoll, NY: Orbis Books, 1998).

## Harris on a Feminist Path to Awakening

Much attention was given by Harris to the significance for women's spiritual awakening of the denigration of women's bodies in society and in religion. She considered awareness and attention to this phenomenon as crucial for women's ongoing awakening process. She rebuked teachings from the past that encouraged women to deny sexual pleasure or suffer abuse in silence:[27] 'Too much spirituality from the past, both in the Eastern and Western worlds, has taught withdrawal from and denial of the body, and even doing violence to the body ... much if not all spirituality is tainted with suggestions that women's bodies are a source of evil, a source of "temptation" into sin.' Awareness is key to changing this, 'at times when women have been unreflective, or have not learned to love themselves first, they have, unfortunately, developed the truly terrible and terrorising capacity for hating themselves and other women.'[28] She asserted that the demon of women hating will need to be exorcised from spirituality as women journey into awakening.

It will be important for women's awakening, Harris insisted, that women grow to love their bodies and to heal the negation of women by their own gender and in society as a whole. Because awakening begins with the senses, it made sense for Harris that, for women, awakening can begin with their bodies; in fact, she asserted that it's the only place to start. She proposed that women might see menstruation as a spiritual gift, a blessing, rather than a curse, offering time for quiet and reflection. Harris also counselled women to be aware of the phases of the moon and corresponding changes in the body.

Harris also criticised spirituality of the past for its equation of the spiritual life with withdrawal from the world, severing connections with family and society. She considered this intolerable for women's spiritual life since women deeply value connection. Citing the work of Carol Gilligan and Nancy Chodorow, whose research concluded that girls commonly

27    Harris, *Dance of the Spirit*, 8.
28    Ibid.

come to understand themselves through relatedness, whereas boys often understand themselves as individual and autonomous;[29] she argued that separation may be seen as a threat by women, while for men intimacy and attachment may feel more threatening.[30]

Nicola Slee, Director of Research at the Queen's Foundation for Ecumenical Theological Education in Birmingham, has more recently highlighted the importance of relational connections for women's spiritual awakening journeys, in her insightful study of the spiritual development of thirty women who were self-designated as Christian or previously Christian. Her research, published in 2004 in *Women's Faith Development: Patterns and Processes*, draws conclusions on this relationality which are in alignment with Harris's theories:

> Their experiences of awakenings through relationships with others ... frequently failed to conform to the stereotypes of the spiritual life which they had received, which prized the flight from the mundane, the denial of the body and the passions and the prioritising of religious ideals over the demands of connection.[31]

To support the awakening process, Harris advised women to adopt certain attitudes and approaches, such as going out without wearing make-up, in order to gain an appreciation of the natural beauty of the face and to present one's self without the mask of make-up to the world. Although she confessed to wearing make-up herself, she argued that it is symbolic of all the masks women wear: 'A much more constricting and damaging mask is the false expression we so often wear: of peaceful agreement when we are in raging disagreement; of pleasure when we are actually disgusted'.[32] Awakening is supported, she asserted, by being true to one's self and not pretending.

She urged women to stop believing in untruths internalised from society and religion which imply that women are weak while men are strong.

---

29    C. Gilligan, *In a Different Voice: Psychological Theory and Women's Development* (Cambridge, MA; London: Harvard University Press, 1982).
30    Harris, *Dance of the Spirit*, 40.
31    N. Slee, *Women's Faith Development: Patterns and Processes*, Explorations in Practical, Pastoral, and Empirical Theology (Aldershot: Ashgate, 2004), 170.
32    Harris, *Dance of the Spirit*, 16.

She acknowledged the devastating effect of what she terms the religious lies women have interiorised, 'that God is male, and so men just understand him (him?) better than women do ... That women are not worthy to serve at the altar of God, even to touch it ... That sin was introduced to the world by a woman'.[33] Her advice on this topic to women was to harbour an attitude of disbelief in those statements and ideas. From the initial awakening women must be willing to grow up, she added, and realise that if one is to be authentic, she will not please everyone or believe all that has been passed on.

Harris drew on the Hebrew teaching on *dabhar*, a Hebrew word with connotes God's creative and redemptive power in the world.[34] According to Harris, this Divine creative power lies within, waiting to be tapped by uncovering or bringing to light what has been in the shadow realms. Letting go of false notions of one's self enables a more truthful sense of being to emerge. This can be achieved by exploring the inner world, befriending what has been revealed and integrating it into the psyche.

Harris noted a common experience in awakening women with whom she had worked, of a sense of a calling from God, from another, or from a social justice issue.[35] Often women become aware of gifts they had neglected and befriend them. They also become aware of their brokenness and the brokenness of the world or face up to the reality of misogyny in society. She stressed that the outcome of this is not despair but the birth of a new wisdom: 'For beneath the brokenness lies a second discovery, critical to spirituality: the power residing within us to face and overcome the brokenness'.[36] A woman discovers her power, her capacities and abilities to deal with the brokenness.

Amongst those abilities, Harris included the power to be vulnerable. Being able to be open about one's limitations reveals a capacity for truth. Thirty years after the book was published, the workplace is still not seen to

---

33   Ibid., 17–18.
34   A. Robinson, *God and the World of Signs: Trinity, Evolution, and the Metaphysical Semiotics of C. S. Peirce* (Leiden; Boston, MA: Brill, 2010), 69.
35   Harris, *Dance of the Spirit*, 31.
36   Ibid., 37.

uphold the women who profess their limitations and their vulnerability. A gender pay gap still exists worldwide. Women are expected to shoulder responsibilities of home-making, mothering as well as their employment, to the detriment of their health and well-being.

The theme of healing women's oppression as a crucial element of the spiritual path will be developed later in respect of the writing of Beverly Lanzetta. Meanwhile, Roberto Assagioli's theory of psychosynthesis, the natural drive in the human person towards spiritual awakening and integration, provides another useful perspective through which to develop a theory of spiritual awakening in women with chronic invisible illness.

## Roberto Assagioli: Psychosynthesis and Spiritual Awakening

A second foundational theorist for this research is Roberto Assagioli (1888–1974). An Italian medical doctor and psychoanalyst and a founder of transpersonal psychology, Assagioli, along with Abraham Maslow (1908–1970), argued for the spiritual nature of the human being. He spent his career developing a theory of psychosynthesis to enable, 'the awakening and manifestation of latent potentialities of the human being'.[37] The term awakening, he explained, 'suggests the perception, the becoming aware of a new area of experience, the opening of hitherto closed eyes to an inner reality previously ignored'.[38] His work has significance for research into chronic illness and spiritual awakening. Although trained in medicine and psychiatry, Assagioli's approach was psycho-spiritual, meaning that the human being in his framework was considered to be a spiritual being having a human experience. Assagioli saw an innate drive towards healing and harmonisation within the human individual, and in relationships. Influenced by the world's great religions, Assagioli viewed psychological

---

37  R. Assagioli, *Psychosynthesis: A Manual of Principles and Techniques* (London: Viking Press, 1971), 38.
38  Ibid., 40.

symptoms and illness not as phenomena to be pathologised and eliminated, but as opportunities for spiritual awakening and personal growth. In 1910 he pioneered his theory of *psychosynthesis* to reflect his recognition and affirmation of what he termed the higher aspects of human nature. Assagioli believed that many symptoms and disturbances come as a result of a person's higher potential calling her forth rather than from trauma in childhood.

This notion has been extended since the time of Assagioli. In psychotherapy Assagioli's model is present in modalities such as *Process Oriented Psychology*, founded by physicist and transpersonal psychoanalyst Arnold Mindell, a former training analyst at the C. G. Jung Institute in Switzerland. Mindell posits that symptoms, be they physical or psychological, are not merely pathologies to be fixed or transcended, but instead are expressions of what is needed for further growth. Working with symptoms using non-judgemental presence in a phenomenological fashion enables awakening and deepening in wisdom. Mindell asserted, 'a symptom is not only a pathological defect in normal health but a "big dream", a huge opportunity and opening to life never experienced before. The more drastic the symptom, the vaster the potential of the given individual'.[39]

Assagioli's iconic oval diagram (see Figure 1) serves to illustrate constituent elements involved in the process of spiritual awakening by clarifying the relationships between the conscious, the unconscious, and the superconscious aspects of the human person. It provides a useful framework for mapping the concept of spiritual awakening.

Significantly for this research, in a 1967 paper on psychosynthesis and the body, Assagioli made clear his belief that mind and body were inseparable, describing the human person as a *psycho-physical* structure. Here he advocated the recognition of the significance of the 'higher' functions, in other words the spiritual dimension of the human being, in physical illnesses conditions.[40]

---

39    A. Mindell, *Dreambody: The Body's Role in Revealing the Self*, 2nd Edition (Portland, Oregon: Lao Tse, 1998), 14.

40    R. Assagioli, 'Psychosynthesis Medicine and Bio-Psychosynthesis', *Psychosynthesis Research Foundation*, no. 21 (1967), <http://www.psykosyntese.dk/a-147/>. Accessed 20 May 2016.

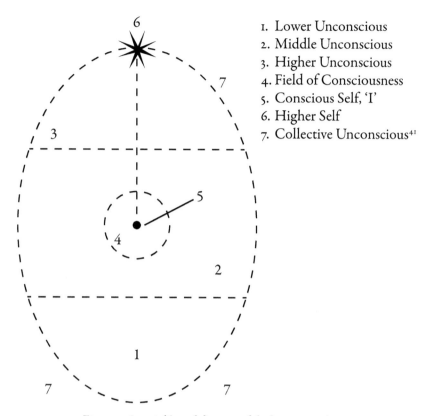

1. Lower Unconscious
2. Middle Unconscious
3. Higher Unconscious
4. Field of Consciousness
5. Conscious Self, 'I'
6. Higher Self
7. Collective Unconscious[41]

Figure 1. Assagioli's oval diagram of the human psyche

## Assagioli and the Awakening of the Higher Self

Roberto Assagioli used the oval diagram to illustrate 'the psychosynthetic conception of the psycho-physical structure of the human being'.[42] The surrounding oval shape represents the whole of the bio-physical human being.

---

41   Psychosynthesis Online, 'Psychosynthesis – Free Clip Art', accessed 3 February 2015, <http://www.psychosynthesisonline.com/psychosynthesis-clip-art.html>.

42   Assagioli, 'Psychosynthesis Medicine and Bio-Psychosynthesis'.

The lower unconscious layer of the oval is where repressed painful memories are stored alongside basic drives. The middle unconscious part holds experiences and memories that are easily accessible. The higher unconscious or superconscious is the realm of transpersonal experience – it is the source of human higher values, of authentic meaning-making, artistic qualities, inspiration, insight and creative awareness. It is what prompts us to humanitarian activities; it is the bearer of our human potential that can be manifested in the future.[43]

Self, referred to also as the *higher Self* or *transpersonal Self*, is a permanent centre and serves as a synthesising force.[44] 'The realisation of the Transpersonal Self is the mark of spiritual fulfilment,' explained Pierro Ferrucci, a psychotherapist and former student of Assagioli.

> Identification with the Transpersonal Self is a rare occurrence – for some individuals the culmination of years of discipline ... It was described in ancient times with the Sanskrit word *sat-chit-ananda*: being-consciousness-bliss. The Transpersonal Self, while retaining a sense of individuality lives at the level of universality, in a realm where personal plans and concerns are overshadowed by the wider vision of the whole.[45]

Transpersonal Self is represented by the star at the top of the diagram. Assagioli emphasised that Self is located at the top merely for convenience as the illustration is not three dimensional – he appreciated that Self is not limited to the higher realms but also located in everyday life and in the depths of the lower unconscious.

The small circle representing the field of consciousness signifies how limited the field of everyday awareness may be, and how the human being is often distanced from the potential experiences of the larger picture, including the gifts of the superconscious. The field of consciousness comprises, 'that part of our personality of which we are directly aware; the incessant

---

43   Assagioli, *Psychosynthesis: A Manual of Principles and Techniques*, 17.
44   Ibid., 19.
45   P. Ferrucci, *What We May Be: The Vision and Techniques of Psychosynthesis* (London: Aquarian Press, 1990), 45.

flow of sensations, images, thoughts, feelings, desires and impulses which we can observe, analyse and judge'.[46]

The 'I', also referred to as the self (with a small s), is the point of pure awareness, the centre of awareness and will. It is located within the personality but connected to the higher Self. 'I' is a reflection of Self, and by growing in awareness and disidentifying with thoughts and feelings, aspects of Self such as empathy, compassion, inspiration, love, altruism, and creativity are more readily available to it.

Assagioli's psychosynthesis ultimately is about uncovering a deeper sense of the human person and the meaning of life for each one. Such knowing emerges with a certain kind of introspection: 'The changing contents of our consciousness (the sensations, thoughts, feelings etc.) are one thing, while the "I", the self, the center of our consciousness is another'.[47] The processes of psychosynthesis help build a relationship with Self which in turn can assist with healing, often affording experiences of states of mystical consciousness, and an opportunity to discern purpose and meaning in life.

Pertinent to the research topic is the brokenness of the line which divides the fields of consciousness. At certain times in life, according to psychosynthesis theory, energies from the higher unconscious, *descendant energies*, enter into the field of consciousness producing spiritual awakening. This can happen following a time of crisis or loss such as illness:

> the bursting in of superconscious elements into the conscious mind in the form of intuitive thoughts, sudden enlightenment or inspiration. Often these are spontaneous, unexpected occurrences, but sometimes they are a response to a call or an invocation on the part of the individual, whether conscious or not.[48]

These spiritual energies are bearers of

---

46   R. Assagioli, *Psychosynthesis: A Collection of Basic Writings* (New York: Penguin Books, 1987), 18.

47   Ibid.

48   R. Assagioli, *Transpersonal Development*, revised edn (Forres: Smiling Wisdom, imprint of Inner Way Productions, 2008), 21.

not only the specific religious experience, but all the states of awareness, all the functions and activities which have as common denominator the possessing of values
higher than the average, values such as the ethical, the esthetic, the heroic, the humanitarian and the altruistic.[49]

Assagioli devised the theory and methods of psychosynthesis to enable
the individual consciously to facilitate the process through which spiritual awakening, healing and integration can take place. However, he also
claimed that psychosynthesis is happening all the time in the life of the
human person as new insights are emerging into the field of consciousness and are being synthesised. It is part of the human maturation process.

It is beyond the scope of this book to discuss all of Assagioli's principles and techniques. His notion of *will*, which occupies a central place
in his thinking, is reviewed here because it provides a useful apparatus for
understanding the way in which spiritual awakening may occur in chronic
invisible illnesses. In addition, Assagioli's theories of *disidentification* and
*subpersonalities*, further ideas with particular relevance for the topic of
spiritual awakening in illness, will be examined.

### Will and Disidentification

In Figure 1, 'I' is the true self, though it is often buried, masked or lost in
childhood wounds. 'I' has two functions, that of awareness and will. Will
is the function of the 'I' that allows the person to direct consciousness to
a particular object. It thus guides the personality. Through working in a
psychosynthetic context, the 'I' becomes distinct from thoughts, feelings
and obsessions. As the 'I' gains freedom, energies from the Self are enabled to flow into it and into the field of consciousness, enabling spiritual
awakening, greater authenticity and a sense of wholeness. A key goal in
psychosynthesis is for the 'I' to become a master of the personality, and a
servant of the Self.

---

49   Assagioli, *Psychosynthesis: A Manual of Principles and Techniques*, 38.

One of the methods in which the 'I' becomes freed is through dis-identification. The human person who is unaware of thoughts and feelings lives at the mercy of those thoughts and feelings. 'I' is identified with painful aspects of the personality and has no freedom. Through working with a skilled therapist who offers empathic listening and through utilising other techniques such as meditation, the person is enabled to become aware of how the 'I' is being taken over by these facets of the personality. Empathic non-judgemental listening is also, significantly, available in support groups for people who are ill. These are sometimes formal gatherings where people meet to discuss issues pertaining to their condition. In the case of chronic invisible illnesses, support groups are usually informal and operate through a grapevine of personal introductions. Friendships evolve between people who have never met face to face, but are often sustained by telephone conversations. Those with invisible illnesses value their support circle which enables their experience of alienation to be acknowledged and the truth of their condition to be recognised and validated. This often has an effect of freeing up their 'I' from feelings of shame and stigmatisation in which they might be trapped as a result of the reality of their experience not being believed and acknowledged.

## Assagioli's Subpersonality Theory

Central to Assagioli's theory is the notion of *subpersonalities*, which can be construed as the roles or functions people have in life – teacher, daughter, student or carer; it is as though there are multiple personalities living inside every human being.[50] Sometimes these internal entities are in conflict with each other, causing a blockage in the sense of harmony and flow for the person. A subpersonality can also be a frozen aspect from the past, for example, the 'frightened child'. The individual may be unaware that unresolved issues from the past can result in the 'I' being trapped in

---

50   Ibid., 74–5.

such energies. Crucial for freedom of the 'I' and the development of will, Assagioli asserted,

> one should become clearly aware of these subpersonalities because this evokes a measure of understanding of the meaning of psychosynthesis, and how it is possible to synthesise these subpersonalities into a larger organic whole without repressing any of their useful traits.[51]

When harmony is restored between two subpersonalities, a sense of peace and wellbeing ensues. When an individual is ill, it is easy to become unconsciously consumed by the identity of the illness. This is evident in the expression 'I am ill' or 'I am depressed'. Disidentification from the ill subpersonality can enable individuals with illness to realise 'I am not this illness', thus freeing up the 'I' from its overwhelming identity with sickness. Disidentification can be facilitated through empathic listening from a friend or counsellor or through meditation, journaling and other therapeutic techniques. Disidentification enables spiritual awakening and growth in wisdom as all the parts become integrated around the unifying centre of the 'I'.

Assagioli credited every subpersonality with having positive traits which need to be placed at the service of the 'I'. In fact the subpersonality can be seen to have its own oval diagram with a higher unconscious and a Self. Working with the subpersonality and learning of its divine essence provides an opportunity for spiritual awakening by releasing those higher energies into the personality. The individual and society as a whole can benefit from the wisdom that can be released upon disidentification with the 'sick person' subpersonality.

It is noteworthy for the research topic in hand that Assagioli warned that spiritual awakening tends to appear following a crisis in one's life. For the person whose life is smooth, there is insufficient attention to matters of Spirit: 'He takes life as it comes and does not worry about the problems of its meaning; he devotes himself to the satisfaction of his personal desires; he seeks enjoyment of the senses and endeavours to become rich and satisfy his ambitions'.[52] If the individual is religious, Assagioli surmised, the religion would be more of the conventional kind, conforming to the requirements of a Church. The person's life is then hit by change, sudden or slow: 'This may take place after a series of disappointments, not infrequently after some emotional shock, such as the loss of a loved relative or a dear friend'.[53] Then the person begins to inquire into the origin and the purpose of life, 'to question, for instance, the meaning of his own sufferings and those of others, and what justification there may be for so many inequalities in the destinies of men'.[54]

The chronic illness experience and its associated losses enable the human being, albeit through harsh circumstances, to disidentify from subpersonalities which are, for example, associated with striving, looking for approval from others, proving one's self in the world or perhaps being the wage earner in the household. This is a time of great loss, but it also enables a freeing up of the 'I'. The 'I' becomes more available for energies from the Self and the higher unconscious to enter into it. This process constitutes an awakening of spiritual consciousness.

It is interesting to note that, in his teaching on the awakening and development of spiritual consciousness, Roberto Assagioli remarked that spiritual consciousness is not the preserve of those who practise religion but that

> a growing number of individuals today are, consciously or not, desperately searching for something more satisfying, more real, than their normal, everyday lives. Many of them have a keen intellect and a down-to-earth attitude, but are unable to find what they need in traditional religion.[55]

It is also noteworthy that, although Assagioli's theory provides a useful conceptual map which can be applied to the spiritual awakening, it lacks reference as to how the woman's journey might differ from that of a man or how awakening might be facilitated through bodywork practice. Though

---

52 Assagioli, *Psychosynthesis: A Manual of Principles and Techniques*, 40.
53 Ibid., 42.
54 Ibid., 41.
55 Assagioli, *Transpersonal Development*, 19.

Assagioli respected symptoms as potential bearers of wisdom, the focus in his writing was on psychological symptoms rather than physical illnesses. Nevertheless he helped to lay foundations for future exploration of the value of physical illness and symptoms as a vehicle for spiritual awakening. Today there exists a burgeoning of body-oriented psychotherapies such as *sensorimotor* psychotherapy created by Patricia Ogden[56] and the previously cited process oriented psychotherapy which is being developed under the guidance of Arnold Mindell and Amy Mindell.[57]

The spiritual journey of women in particular will now addressed by exploring the work of Beverly Lanzetta whose interpretation of the lives of the women mystics offers another lens through which to view the topic of spiritual awakening in illness.

## Beverly Lanzetta on Spiritual Awakening

My third foundational theorist is Beverly Lanzetta who is a former Professor of Religion of Villanova University, Pennsylvania. Her work combines scholarship in world religions and texts with the study of mysticism and feminist consciousness. Her 2005 book, *Radical Wisdom: A Feminist Mystical Theology*, developed a socially contextualised understanding of spiritual awakening and demonstrated an intense awareness and concern about the suppression of women in different world religions, as well as its consequences for the position of women in society as a whole, and their health. Her feminist mystical theology can illuminate the suffering, trauma and potential spiritual growth of women with invisible illness. She acknowledged the relationship between women's social status and their health, seeing their inner lives as frequently mirroring their personal and

---

56   P. Ogden, *Trauma and the Body: A Sensorimotor Approach to Psychotherapy*, 1st edn (New York: W. W. Norton & Company, 2006).

57   A. Mindell, *Metaskills: The Spiritual Art of Therapy* (Portland, OR: Lao Tse Press, 2003).

collective health.[58] Her observations about the process and the circumstances of spiritual awakening of women can be usefully applied to women today who have chronic invisible illnesses.

In particular Lanzetta has developed the concept of the *feminine dark night* within the framework of *Via Feminina*. Building on the work of Constance Fitzgerald, she argues that the prejudice against women in religion and society constitutes an attack on woman's nature because the distinctiveness of female sexuality represents the way the divine is embodied in womanhood. She proposes that women, in order to heal and become empowered, need to address those wounds.

She has studied the medieval women mystics and has re-read their material through a feminist lens. She has explored the processes they used to 'name, eliminate, and transform their soul suffering, and to dignify and empower themselves as women'.[59] Lanzetta considers the journey to awakening the soul as not only necessary for women to heal, but also for healing the subjugation of women worldwide as, 'What harms a woman's soul reverberates in her physical, emotional and mental spheres, generating suffering in every area of her life'.[60]

This healing journey is not exclusively for women, she emphasised; the integration of the feminine aspect in the male is as necessary as the reclaiming by women of their masculine energy. She has been influenced by Thomas Merton who had already proposed that by healing the internal split in themselves, people help to heal division in the whole world. For Lanzetta, the suppression of the female mirrors the most fundamental tensions such as, 'ancient division in intellectual history between body and soul, matter and spirit, human and divine, humanity and the natural world'.[61] This division, she has argued, is responsible for violence against women and other subjugated groups. She has gone as far as asserting that this wound 'is at the core of our cultural pathology'.[62]

---

58   Lanzetta, *Radical Wisdom*, 9.
59   Ibid., 2.
60   Ibid.
61   Ibid., 10–11.
62   Ibid.

Lanzetta has drawn on the writings of Pseudo-Dionysius, a sixth-century Syrian theologian and philosopher, who described two types of contemplative consciousness, the positive or *cataphatic* and the negative *apophatic*, to advance her argument. The positive path involves the use of names and symbols for God, prayer and activity, whereas the negative path or *via negativa* denotes the leaving behind of all images of God and entering into *nothingness*. Lanzetta's reflections about the path of negation may be applied to the phenomenon of spiritual awakening through illness and its bedfellow, isolation: 'The corollary to the negation of concepts is the unsaying, undoing, and unwilling of the "lower self" – that entity defined by the world of attraction, ego demand and economy – to find the one thing necessary, the true self'.[63] The process of chronic illness may present for women an opportunity 'to leave behind societal and often anti-female views to gain dignity, power and self-worth'.[64]

Lanzetta believes that women's health is affected by the suppression of women in society. She noted that, according to the United Nations Fourth World Conference on Women, there is still no country in the world where men and women enjoy full equality.[65] She argued that women's dignity cannot be segregated from 'the exterior state of our global community where women are still the most oppressed of oppressed groups.'[66] Suppression of women in the spheres of religion and society as a whole, Lanzetta has argued, is violence directed at the core of a woman's nature, her female sexuality represents the way the divine is embodied in womanhood, and an attack on female sexuality is an attack on her embodiment of the divine in the world.[67] Lanzetta proposed that the mystical journey, as charted by the Spanish mystic Teresa of Avila in the sixteenth century, and her collaborator, St John of the Cross, could be reinterpreted for today as a map to gain inner freedom.

63    Ibid., 15.
64    Ibid., 19.
65    Ibid., 1.
66    Ibid., 10.
67    Ibid., 2.

## Teresa of Avila: Surveyor of the Soul's Journey

Lanzetta concluded that healing internalised misogyny constituted a core product of the contemplative path for mystic St Teresa of Avila (1515–1582). Teresa was a Carmelite nun, a writer and teacher of mysticism. She reformed the Carmelite order in Spain and, in 1970, became the first woman in the Roman Catholic world to earn the title Doctor of the Church. Lanzetta has created a unique overview of the journey of awakening from the 1577 chronicle of the Spanish mystic entitled *Las Moradas* [*The Interior Castle*].[68] This classical record of the mystical life was based on Teresa's own experience and attends to the psychological dimensions of the journey towards union with God, in the language of her day.

Teresa applied a metaphor to the mystical journey of an interior crystalline castle with seven dwellings through which the person passes before reaching an advanced stage of union with the divine. The journey is one of progression from a sense of wretchedness to self-dignity. The first three rooms deal with human striving for a greater sense of self. The fourth room, a transitional space of awakening in preparation for entry to the final three rooms in this crystalline castle, bears particular relevance to this study.

John Welch, who holds the chair of Carmelite Studies at the Washington Theological Union, has explored the parallels between Carl Jung's thinking on individuation of the self, and the journey of Teresa of Avila through the rooms of her interior castle. Teresa's journey, he argued, 'is an inward journey towards God which is, at the same time, a movement into self-knowledge.'[69] His publication *Spiritual Pilgrims: Carl Jung and Teresa of Avila*[70] (1982) divides Teresa's movement through the castle into two phases of the individuation progress. The transition point between the two phases is the fourth room. Due to the fourth room's relevance to this research topic, this part of Welch's discourse is worth quoting at length:

---

68    K. Kavanaugh, *The Interior Castle Study Edition*, reprint edn (Washington, DC: ICS Publications, 2010).

69    J. Welch, *Spiritual Pilgrims: Carl Jung and Teresa of Avila*, 1st edn (New York: Paulist Press, 1982), 3.

70    Ibid.

The first phase involved the first three dwelling places. The second phase begins
in the fourth dwelling place and continues through the remaining three dwelling
places. The first three dwelling places are characterized by outer preoccupations,
while the last three have a definite inner orientation. The first phase is active and
controlling. The second phase is receptive and letting go. The fourth dwelling place
marks the transition from outer to inner and signals the deep interior work of the
individuation process.[71]

Welch likens the first phase or three rooms in Teresa's castle to adolescence,
and the last phase to more mature years: 'In terms of the life-cycle the first
three dwelling places could reflect the years from adolescence, where an
initial conversion and choice of vocation usually takes place, to the midlife years where a "second conversion" is needed'.[72]

In the first room the soul is absorbed in daily affairs, image and possessions.[73] There is little interest in prayer and even less in self-reflection. Teresa
wrote about this phase thus: 'it is a shame and unfortunate that through
our own fault we don't understand ourselves or know who we are'.[74] For
the purposes of this research, this is the pre-illness phase in the life of a
woman before becoming chronically ill. Assagioli's subpersonality theory
contributes a useful insight: it could be said that the individual is identified
with a career-woman aspect of her psyche, attending to the needs of the
ego. She may be attached to earning a living, having an impressive career,
or being a mother and responding to the demands of everyday life. The idea
is that in the first room there is little time or attention for the inner life.

The second room, progressing inward towards the centre, is where,
after the first steps have been taken in reflectiveness, the person is receptive to insights from a deeper source of wisdom. A call from God is heard.
Here, Teresa finds that hearing the call to growth is difficult as a person
becomes alert to human brokenness and inner conflicts. Teresa explained
that a call from God can emanate from a variety of sources including illness and hardship:

71    Ibid., 97.
72    Ibid., 98.
73    Lanzetta, *Radical Wisdom*, 106.
74    Kavanaugh, *The Interior Castle Study Edition*, 34.

through words spoken by other good people, or through sermons, or through what is read in good books, or through the many things that are heard and by which God calls, or through illnesses and trials, or also through a truth that he teaches during the brief moments we spend in prayer; however lukewarm these moments may be, God esteems them.[75]

For the purposes of this study, the second room concerns the onset of illness and its accompanying traumas. Illness is the event that disrupts everyday life. Aristotle named such disruptive events in life as the *peripeteia*, the unexpected event that changes everything for the tragic hero. In this study, the second room presents an illness from which there is no return to life as it was. It is often the occasion where the individual calls on a higher source of power. The illness usually forces people to face their shadow side during long hours spent in isolation.

Teresa allocated the third room to those who strive to lead a virtuous life; but they are still sufficiently attached to worldly interests that they are in danger of regressing. Life is under control in a spiritual and social sense, but that very control and the stasis it brings can lead to spiritual numbness or even a type of fundamentalism. For this study, in the third room, people with chronic illness still attempt to hold on to stability and to the certainties of life as it was before illness descended. In the case of women with invisible illnesses, there is, perhaps, still a dependency on finding a cure within the dominant cultural medical paradigm.

The fourth room, located in the middle of the seven, is a transitional stage between the first three rooms and the last three. It is the room where awakening occurs and where a contemplative stance begins. Welch has averred that this is the room in which the inner journey has truly begun.

> The individual's persona-identification has cracked and ego-consciousness no longer has total control of the psyche. A new, more powerful center is emerging which calls attention to itself and demands a response.[76]

75 Ibid.
76 Welch, *Spiritual Pilgrims*, 104.

For those who are chronically ill with a stigmatised illness, circumstances of loss and isolation facilitate the cracking of the ego-consciousness to which Welch refers. The fourth room is the transition space where surrender happens accompanied by a degree of acceptance of the illness. A sense of calm often enters the psyche.

As observed, Welch's theory on Avila's interior castle notes that the second phase, from the fourth room through to the sixth, concerns the deep interior work of the individuation process, in contrast to the first three rooms which are more to do with adaptation to changed life circumstances. In the case of this study, the journey through the second phase may be facilitated by conversations with other people with similar illnesses who are travelling a similar interior path.

In Teresa's model, there is a deep openness to transcendent wisdom in the fifth dwelling and a quieting of resistance to circumstances. The sixth dwelling is the locus of a deeper appreciation and embracing of the changed circumstances in life, and the seventh, located at the centre, symbolises commitment to living within a renewed horizon. Lanzetta elucidated, 'As the soul advances towards the center of its castle, consciousness moves from oppression to freedom, from human love to divine love, and from doubt to certainty'.[77]

Mystics such as Teresa of Avila and John of the Cross lived their entire mystical journey within a strong theistic worldview. This is not necessarily the case with all people who are ill. Nevertheless, parallels can be drawn between the mystical path and the journey of growth in illness. Therefore, the conceptual framework of their mystical path can be applied to spiritual awakening in chronic illness. Whilst the desire of the ill person is not explicitly to unite with a divine figure, there is a deep desire for healing, for meaning, for resolution of the chaos, for peace, for understanding and love. These qualities constitute attributes of the higher unconscious and of the Self in Assagioli's psychosynthesis theory. A call for healing therefore may be viewed as a call or an invocation to an ultimate healing power in the universe.

---

77    Lanzetta, *Radical Wisdom*, 108.

In practical terms, Teresa of Avila gained freedom as a woman by walking the mystical path. The era of the Inquisition presented life-threatening challenges for women mystics. She suffered ridicule and intimidation by members of the clergy who, fearful of contemplative practice as a threat to non-experiential Christian teaching, or fearful of being suspected of heresy themselves, accused her of consorting with the devil.[78] The revolutionary vernacular theology of Meister Eckhart and the Beguines which had affirmed women's awakening and mystical experiences in northern Europe in the thirteenth to fourteenth centuries was not available to support Teresa, owing to the prevailing socio-political landscape where literature on mysticism was banned.[79]

Teresa felt deprived of a confessor, or spiritual director, who could understand and support her inner journey. She had tried many spiritual directors before she found John of the Cross and complained in her memoirs that great harm had been done to her by some of them whom she had approached. Her spiritual directors did not understand the nature or the fullness of a woman's spiritual journey; she complained that: 'half-learned confessors have done my soul great harm when I have been unable to find a confessor with as much learning as I like'.[80] Regarding the Church's obsession with the devil she wrote, 'without doubt, I fear those who have such great fear of the devil more than I do the devil himself, for he cannot do anything to me. Whereas these others, especially if they are confessors, cause severe disturbance; I have undergone now some years of such great trial that I am amazed now at how I was able to suffer it'.[81] In 1567 she met John of the Cross while she was setting up her second reformed Carmelite convent. Initially John had been Teresa's student, to whom she taught an appreciation of her sisters' way of life in order that he would have a clear

---

78 Ibid., 110.
79 Peter Tyler, theologian at St Mary's University, Twickenham, has presented an examination of Teresa's work in the context of the Spanish Inquisition: P. Tyler, *Teresa of Avila: Doctor of the Soul* (London: Bloomsbury Academic, 2014).
80 K. Kavanaugh and O. Rodriguez, *Teresa of Avila: The Book of Her Life* (Indianapolis, IN: Hackett, 2008), 19.
81 Ibid., 171.

understanding of it, and so that his spiritual direction work with them would be enhanced.[82]

The inner strength and sense of self-worth gained by Teresa through progressing along the path of mystical wisdom gave her tremendous courage and determination to write about and to teach her version of contemplation in sixteenth-century Inquisitional Spain. With skill and bravery, she proceeded to write and to teach what she had learned experientially. Teresa's journey convinced Lanzetta that the mystic's path had a lot to offer women who suffer from oppression today, 'this mystical emptiness of self initiates an unreserved responsibility in which our mystics reclaim their dignity as women and articulate a new feminine way of liberation for themselves and for others'.[83]

Teresa's journey was marked by long bouts of physical illness and pain throughout her life and her insights about pain and loss offer a useful paradigm for those who are ill today. She considered pain and joy as not opposed to each other, but as two aspects of drawing closer to the deep mystery of life.[84] Her struggle with feelings of unworthiness mirrors the journey of many women who are chronically ill who look to their interior world to find healing. She felt alienated in a Church where she had been ridiculed for presenting a woman's version of the mystic journey. She complained that a critical element of women's spiritual struggles was left out of Church teachings. She was aware that 'women's self-doubt and self-loathing not only were a result of personal failings but were formed also by deep social and religious roots'.[85] Lanzetta has viewed Teresa's particular struggle with her self-loathing, with its religious roots, as Teresa's version of what St John of the Cross had termed the *dark night of the soul*.

Teresa of Avila conceived of the spiritual life as one in which the person must learn to detach from the temporary attractions of the good life through determination and practice in order to experience a higher order of freedom

82    Ibid., xxiii.
83    Lanzetta, *Radical Wisdom*, 118.
84    Ibid., 117.
85    Ibid., 124.

and happiness.[86] Detachment is facilitated in illness, however, as the ego is robbed of its attachments in the world of career and competitiveness. Long days of isolation in chronic illness provide many of the conditions such as loss and solitude, which are favourable for the awakening process, precipitating a shift in perspective: 'This emphasis on "being" over "doing" is one of degree, a shift in perspective that allows the person to move from a deeper center than the one normally demanded by the world'.[87]

Women who experience chronic illness, unlike many mystics, have not set out with a desire for solitude; rather it has been foisted upon them with all of the other losses that illness brings. Nevertheless, the proliferation of art, poetry, narratives of illness and support groups of people who are ill would suggest that their illness has brought about an awakening to a new dimension of consciousness.

### Illness as Apophatic Experience: Insights from John of the Cross

Carmelite friar John of the Cross (1542–1591), according to Lanzetta, provided the finest clarification of the nature of the *via negativa* or *apophatic* experience. Lanzetta has offered the experiential knowledge of the dark night of the soul gained by John and Teresa as a conceptual framework to explore 'when the soul of a woman turns inward to heal her deep divide and to claim her equality'.[88] Lanzetta's observations offer rich material for the exploration of the phenomenon of spiritual awakening in women with chronic invisible illnesses.

John of the Cross termed the soul's passage of awakening, from attachment to worldly attractions to union with God, *una noche oscura*, a dark night. The three reasons he offered for labelling it thus were: the passage involved releasing the desire for worldly possessions, whether physical, mental, emotional or spiritual; secondly it involved faith, which for the intellect is a dark night; finally, it entailed opening to God's transcendent

---

86    Ibid., 109.
87    Ibid., 33.
88    Ibid., 120.

wisdom, an inflow and an illumination and an infusion which can also appear like a dark night to the human being.

To John, the dark night is necessarily desolate for it has the job of releasing the identity of the soul as a new being: 'St John's usage of the term "dark night" implies a confrontation with *nada* (nothing) and signifies the critical transition each person makes across the frozen pond of human ego to the liquid waters of liberation and intimacy'.[89] His brutal incarceration in 1577 for nine months, by a group of confrere Carmelites who challenged his efforts to reform the order, influenced the development of his *dark night* theology. The humiliating and painful public lashings in front of his community, and the isolation he experienced whilst imprisoned in a small cell, all provided external traumas, or a 'purgatory' for the soul.[90]

In John's theology of the soul, he considered the soul as having two parts. The lower soul, or the sensory soul, is turned towards the body, and the higher soul is turned in the direction of spiritual matters. John wrote of a twofold dark night, the dark night of the senses (lower soul) and the dark night of the spirit (higher soul).

Table 1. Dark night

|  | Senses/Lower Soul (sensory attachments purged) | Spirit/Higher Soul (spiritual attachments purified) |
|---|---|---|
| Active | Person is pro-active in controlling senses, e.g. searching for likeminded communities, meditation practices, prayer, healing Masses, yoga, holy wells | Purification of the spirit and the presence of Sophia, the figure of Wisdom |
| Passive | God is in charge and grants the person relief from attachments and worldly desires and places her in a state of contemplation | God heals the soul of its suffering with a special infusion of divine love |

---

89    Ibid., 121.
90    K. Kavanaugh and E. Larkin, eds, *John of the Cross: Selected Writings*, new edn (New York: Paulist Press, 1988), 206.

Lanzetta emphasised though that this is a realm of 'forsakenness and emptiness', where, 'the soul is lifted above the three faculties of memory, understanding and will to pass over to a dark and incomprehensible union with God.' Although the person feels abandoned by God during the dark night, John stressed that 'the soul is being raised up to an illumination so bright it appears dark to the disordered and suffering spirit.' Therefore the dark night is that night 'more lovely than dawn'.[91]

Constance Fitzgerald, a Carmelite theologian who has devoted much of her intellectual life to the interpretation of the work of St John of the Cross, offered an explication of the dark night which applies to the experience of awakening in the case of those with invisible illnesses:

> At the deepest levels of night, in a way one could not have imagined it could happen, one sees the withdrawal of all one has been certain of and depended upon for reassurance and affirmation .... All supports seem to fail one, and only the experience of emptiness, confusion, isolation, weakness, loneliness, and abandonment remains. In the frantic search for reassurance, one wonders if anyone – friend or spouse or God – is really 'for me', is trustworthy. But no answer is given to the question.[92]

The fruits of owning one's powerlessness and poverty enable the person to leave the world of rejection, leading to an awakening to a new level of solidarity and compassion. Fitzgerald added:

> Only an experience like this, coming out of the soul's night, brings about the kind of solidarity and compassion that changes the 'I' into a 'we', enabling one to say, 'we poor', 'we oppressed', 'we exploited'. The poor are objects until we are poor, too. This kind of identification with God's people, with the 'other', is the fruit of dark night.[93]

91  Lanzetta, *Radical Wisdom*, 122.

92  C. Fitzgerald, 'Impasse and Dark Night', in *Women's Spirituality: Resources for Christian Development*, ed. J. Wolski Conn (New York: Paulist Press, 1988), secs 287–311, pp. 297–8.

93  Ibid., 298.

## Lanzetta's Via Feminina

Beverly Lanzetta has proposed that the thinking of John of the Cross and of Teresa of Avila had emerged out of a religious worldview characterised by sin-based theology and thus their writing could lack appeal for many spiritual seekers today. She recommends a new mysticism that resonates with women today, stripped of patriarchal overtones.[94] She argues that Christian mysticism had been a product of a patriarchal world view and that the traditional path of the mystic must be augmented for our time to confront injustices toward the feminine.[95] Constance Fitzgerald has, in a similar manner, broadened the concept of the dark night from the cloisters to connote impasse in its broader social context. Every human being experiences impasse or dark night, societies experience it, those on diverse spiritual paths experience it, and indeed spirituality itself also experiences it.

Fitzgerald has argued that impasse or dark night is a condition of stagnation which defies fixing with the logical rational mind. Human beings encounter impasse in life, as does society as a whole. She suggested that women's spirituality is in a state of impasse. The old patriarchal images of God no longer work, but no satisfactory image or structure has come into being. This is a time to yield to the impasse, 'responding with full consciousness of one's suffering in the impasse yet daring to believe that new possibilities, beyond immediate vision, can be given'.[96] Illness can provide suitable terrain, with its losses, suffering and isolation, for responding with such full consciousness to one's suffering. Its impasse can be the condition for creative growth and transformation under certain circumstances,

> if the limitations of one's humanity and human condition are squarely faced and the sorrow of finitude allowed to invade the human spirit with real, existential powerlessness; if the ego does not demand understanding in the name of control and predictability but is willing to admit the mystery of its own being and surrender itself to

94   Lanzetta, *Radical Wisdom*, 12.
95   Ibid., 17.
96   Fitzgerald, 'Impasse and Dark Night', 289–90.

this mystery; if the path into the unknown, into the uncontrolled and unpredictable margins of life, is freely taken when the path of deadly clarity fades.[97]

Fitzgerald has opined that a key challenge women face is to engage with the infinite mystery of life through the apophatic path which involves contemplation, spiritual conversation, and the revision of inherited frameworks. This will lead to a new frontier in spirituality: 'If the impasse in which feminists find themselves is dark night, then a new experience of God, transformative of alienating symbols, is already breaking through even though it is not comprehensible yet, and impasse is a call to development, transcendence, new life, and understanding.'[98]

Lanzetta has developed the concept of the *feminine dark night* within the framework of 'Via Feminina'. Building on the work of Constance Fitzgerald, she proposes a feminist mystical theology of healing for women by adding another passage of the soul which she terms the *via feminina* which would add to the framework of the dark night of the soul offered by John of the Cross.[99] This is a type of via negativa, apophasis or undoing, a negation, or a criticism of patriarchy in the lives and interactions of women and men. It encompasses a period of letting go of untruths about women, followed by a period of reintegration of spiritual wisdom and soul healing. She argues that women benefit from such a healing process that moves them from oppression and illness to liberation and healing.

Teresa herself went through this experience and although she did not label it explicitly as a stage on the journey, this was inferred in her writing. The via feminina, 'specifically locates a woman's struggle to achieve fullness of being within her soul's internalisation of misogyny particular to her world and God's suffering of the violation of womanhood.'[100] Teresa dealt with the cruel behaviour meted out to her in a male-dominated Church and felt the pain of female embodiment, but her gift in return was an inflow

97  Ibid., 290–1.
98  Fitzgerald, 'Impasse and Dark Night'.
99  Lanzetta, *Radical Wisdom*, 16.
100  Ibid., 125.

of divine wisdom. She gained the strength to understand this cruelty as a 'desecration of the holy'.[101]

Lanzetta has charted three stages of Teresa's via feminina, each of which bear strong resonances in women with chronic invisible illnesses who have felt alienated from friends, the medical profession and the religion of their upbringing. First of all Teresa suffered alienation from herself, her friends and her interests, and confronted both her lack of confidence and her view of herself as inferior because of her gender. In the second phase, she suffered alienation from God because of her feelings of unworthiness and a belief that as a woman she wasn't entitled to be intimate with God. The third phase of the via feminina for Teresa, by then an older woman, involved suffering humiliation and cruelty as clergy accused her of consorting with the devil.

In the midst of experiencing profound abandonment in her own Church, however, Teresa felt total encouragement from God. Those experiences empowered her to take a stand for what she believed and, in the frightening atmosphere of the Inquisition, she boldly proceeded to teach her ideas on the mystical path and to speak out for the rights of women and girls.[102] She gained the courage to teach her sisters to value the mystical life over ecclesiastical authority. Demonstrating that the mystical journey is a powerful force for social transformation, the women created new spiritual lineages which were to 'champion mystical practices that fostered the transformation of the social and ecclesial order'.[103]

Teresa had tried to transcend the pain of being a woman. She learned however that, 'woman is not able to reject, or suppress, or mystically override her soul's wounds, but is compelled to feel them at a deeper level and to bear them until they bring forth the birth of her full humanity'.[104]

Significantly, Lanzetta criticises what she refers to as corporate forms of oppression in the medical world where a model of Cartesian reductionism is applied to illnesses which are ultimately connected with women's

---

101   Ibid.
102   Ibid., 126.
103   Ibid., 138.
104   Ibid., 132.

position in the world. Such a model often does not recognise gender differ-ence implications in illnesses and labels women's ailments as psychosomatic or trivialises them.[105] She proposes that an understanding by the medical profession of the journey of the dark night of the feminine would benefit women and society.

This interior process whereby a woman consciously or unconsciously experiences the effects of the violation of her body and spirit as female, becomes an essential precursor to her healing and a positive resource in combating illness, pain, suffering, and dying. The appropriation of the term *dark night* in mental health challenging situations is spreading in the popular media.[106] The term *dark night of the feminine* helps health profes-sionals to realise that even though the causes and conditions of illness may be inscrutable or unknown, the light of wisdom is a powerful healing resource in women's freedom of being and soul healing.[107]

This necessity for woman to enter deeply into suffering in order to heal it is to be found in mythology too, according to Maureen Murdock, the final theorist chosen to elucidate women's awakening to spiritual consciousness.

## Spiritual Awakening and the Heroine's Journey: Maureen Murdock

Maureen Murdock is author of the popular book, *The Heroine's Journey: Woman's Quest for Wholeness*, which was penned in 1990 in response to Joseph Campbell's *The Hero with a Thousand Faces* (1949).[108] A renowned

---

105　B. Lanzetta, 'Women, Soul Wounds, and Integrative Medicine', in *Integrative Women's Health*, eds V. Maizes and T. Low Dog (Oxford: Oxford University Press, 2010), 91.

106　<http://www.drjudithorloff.com/Free-Articles/Suicide-Perspective.htm>. Accessed 18 October 2015.

107　Lanzetta, 'Women, Soul Wounds, and Integrative Medicine', 93.

108　J. Campbell, *The Hero with a Thousand Faces*, Bollingen Series; 17 (New York: Pantheon Books, 1949).

scholar of mythology, Campbell had sketched the hero's journey, discussing the theme of the mythic journey of adventure and transformation that crops up in so many of the great universal myths, for example Homer's epic about the adventures of Odysseus.[109] Campbell outlined the archetypal journey as:

> A hero ventures forth from the world of common day into a region of supernatural wonder: fabulous forces are there encountered and a decisive victory is won: the hero comes back from this mysterious adventure with the power to bestow boons on his fellow man.[110]

The three rites of passage undergone by the hero Campbell identified as separation, initiation and return. Maureen Murdock, however, argues that Campbell's model did not satisfactorily fit the psycho-spiritual journey of women and in 1990 launched her own book in which she developed her prototype of the heroine's journey. Murdock's challenge is not a scholarly work of mythology; she lays out her argument in a popular book in the self-help genre. I have chosen to include it here because her highlighting of the woman's need to acknowledge the wounded feminine in order to awaken spiritually is based on her experience as a psychotherapist. In addition, Murdock's argument illuminates how illness may be construed as a carrier of possibilities for spiritual awakening by providing the circumstances in which this wounding may be addressed.

Murdock's characterisation of women and men is frequently homogenous and, though written in 1990, it is incongruously reminiscent of second-wave feminist theory. Nevertheless, her contribution to the discourse is creative and constitutes a valuable input to theory.

Murdock's model encompasses, like that of Beverly Lanzetta, a descent into pain: 'It may involve seemingly endless periods of wandering, grief and rage ... of looking for lost pieces of herself and meeting the dark feminine.'[111]

Murdock asserts that society is *androcentric*, meaning that it sees the world from a male perspective.[112] The term is associated with American

---

109  Ibid., 58.
110  Ibid., 30.
111  M. Murdock, *The Heroine's Journey* (Boston, MA; New York: Shambhala, 1990), 8.
112  Ibid., 13.

feminist sociologist Charlotte Perkins Gilman (1860–1935) who penned *Our Androcentric Culture* in 1911. Androcentric theory holds the view that man is primary and woman secondary, that all things centre on the male: 'All human standards have been based on male characteristics, and when we wish to praise the work of a woman, we say "she has a masculine mind"'.[113] As a psychotherapist, Murdock recalled that she had heard so often from women clients:

> a resounding cry of dissatisfaction with the successes won in the marketplace. This dissatisfaction is described as a sense of sterility, emptiness, and dismemberment, even a sense of betrayal. These women have embraced the stereotypical male heroic journey and have attained academic, artistic or financial success, yet for many the question remains, 'What is all this for?'[114]

Murdoch argued that these women hadn't travelled far enough on the road of liberation. Their model of success was a masculine one, and it did not satisfy their needs to be whole persons. They had rejected their feminine nature which is conceived of as inferior and dependent in the dominant culture: 'Everything is geared to getting the job done, climbing the academic or corporate ladder; achieving prestige, position, and financial equity; and feeling powerful in the world. This is a heady experience for the heroine, and it is fully supported by our materialistic society, which places supreme value on what you do'.[115]

### Murdock and Mythology

Murdock assessed numerous myths such as that of the celebrated romantic Greek legend of Psyche and Eros. In the story, Psyche, goddess of the soul, falls in love with Eros, god of love. The tale takes many twists and turns, including a trip for Psyche to Hades, the underworld, before she can be united with Eros.

---

113 C. Perkins Gilman, *Our Androcentric Culture* (New York: Charlton Co., 1911), 21.
114 Murdock, *The Heroine's Journey*, 1.
115 Ibid., 6.

Murdock gleaned that the descent to the underworld is about reclaiming the rejected feminine aspect and that the stage cannot be rushed. She considered it as a reclaiming of the Goddess, and argued that the women who undertake reclamation of the rejected feminine are rediscovering the lost soul of their culture.[116] Murdock believed that a woman's task at this stage of our cultural development is to heal the split, 'that tells us that our knowings, wishes, and desires are not as important nor as valid as those of the dominant male culture.' She added that women must gain the courage, 'to live with paradox, the strength to hold the tension of not knowing the answers, and the willingness to listen to our inner wisdom and the wisdom of the planet which begs for change'.[117] Women with chronic invisible illnesses who feel marginalised by the medical profession often develop these traits and abilities as well as concern for the environment. Some make efforts to bring the wisdom that they have gained about the negative effects of chemicals and electro-pollution into the public arena.

Murdock provided a map of the circuitous route a woman takes in order to become a spiritual warrior. The movement is spiral, a continuous process of growth and descent. The first phase of her journey happens at a young age as she rejects her feminine self. Murdock marked this phase as the 'separation from the feminine'.[118] This can occur because she perceives her mother or women in general to be weak. She loses her feminine self and merges with the masculine in order to feed her need to feel powerful. Later in life, having achieved material success, the woman begins to feel betrayed as she experiences emptiness and dissatisfaction with her successes in the world.[119] Though she has gained many valuable qualities in the pursuit of the treasure such as discipline, direction and a certain type of power in her drive to measure up and achieve by male-defined standards, she may feel that she is never good enough: 'Yes, she gained success,

116   Ibid., 9.
117   Ibid., 11.
118   Ibid., 13.
119   Ibid., 5.

independence, and autonomy, but she may have lost a piece of her heart and soul in the process'.[120]

The pain of this experience is the dark night of the feminine, which shares many of the traits of the illness journey. The dark night is terrifying, she warned, but it is important to stick with it, because where there is fear there is power, like the power gained by Teresa of Avila to take a stand for her contemplative teachings.

> It may take weeks, months or years, and for many it may involve a time of voluntary isolation – a period of darkness and silence and of learning the art of deeply listening once again to self: of being instead of doing. The outer world may see this as a depression and a period of stasis. Family, friends, and work associates implore our heroine to 'get on with it'.[121]

*Instinctual Wisdom*

As a consequence of relegating the feminine to an inferior position, Murdock contended, the woman rejects her instinctual body wisdom and, 'when they begin to ignore their bodies they begin to discredit their intuition in favour of their minds'.[122] This issue, when put together with a young woman's unease about her emerging sexuality, often results in a split between body and mind. For Murdock, this was synonymous with repression of their spirituality: 'Women access their spirituality through movement and body awareness, so a denial of the body inhibits the heroine's spiritual development. She ignores her intuition and dreams and pursues the safer activities of the mind'.[123]

Echoing Lanzetta, and the women mystics, Murdock saw the societal consequences of the oppression of women in religious institutions,

120   Ibid., 74.
121   Ibid., 8.
122   Ibid., 24.
123   Ibid.

rejection of the female body, which in our culture has its origins in the Old Testament portrayal of Eve as seductress, has been reinforced in male-dominated religions by taboos about female sexuality for over five thousand years. A woman's gender has been used as an excuse to exclude her from power by political as well as religious institutions.[124]

In order to be ready for her spiritual awakening, Murdock maintained, the heroine must sacrifice false notions of what it means to be heroic. She must find the courage to realise that she is good enough exactly as she is and in doing so she touches into the deeper forces that are the source of her life: 'She becomes real, open, vulnerable, and receptive to a true spiritual awakening'.[125] Saying *no* to the tyranny of expectations from within herself and from society is excruciating in itself, Murdock argued: 'The alternative seen to heroism is self-indulgence, passivity, and lack of importance. That spells death and despair in this culture; our culture supports the path of acquisition, more, better, faster'.[126] The heroine may feel invisible and anything but a heroine.

In the case of women with invisible illnesses, the sense of invisibility is intensified. Often the woman is forced to give up her career and is stripped of her identity due to illness; it doesn't come from choice on a conscious level. She feels acutely the invisibility to which Murdock refers, but she also feels invisible in relation to her illness. Not believed by the medical profession which up to now she has had no reason to distrust, she feels abandoned by the world. The gift involved in this loss is a possibility of a descent into the dark night. Citing a popular book by another feminist author, Sylvia Brenton Perera,[127] Murdock referred to this as *a descent to the Goddess*. Illness, and especially invisible illness with its concomitant feelings of loss of trust, betrayal, rejection and shame, can become that transition period, a period of chaos, 'of losing the way, of being lost in the

---

124  Ibid., 26.
125  Ibid., 69.
126  Ibid., 83.
127  S. Perera, *Descent to the Goddess: A Way of Initiation for Women*, 1st edn (Toronto: Inner City Books, 1981).

forest for some time before we get through and find our path again'.[128] 'A life threatening illness or accident', she proposed, 'the loss of self-confidence or livelihood, a geographical move ... or a broken heart can open the space for dismemberment and descent'.[129] Like Lanzetta, Murdock saw this descent into the depths as a sacred journey; she lamented that it is often viewed in our society as depression which must be medicated and eliminated.[130]

Maureen Murdock emphasised that the dark night is a time when a woman can get to know herself: This is a time when a woman can perhaps for the first time, acquaint herself with, 'her body, her emotions, her sexuality, her intuition, her images, her values, and her mind'.[131] After reclaiming the lost feminine archetype, the heroine can internalise the skills she gained on the path of the masculine warrior and integrate with her newly discovered feminine wisdom. This is the sacred marriage: 'The heroine comes to understand the dynamics of her feminine and masculine nature and accepts them both together'.[132] The outcome of the sacred marriage is the divine child, a sense of wholeness. The heroine 'has gained wisdom from her experiences; she no longer needs to blame the other; she is the other. She brings that wisdom back to share with the world. And the women, men and children of the world are transformed by her journey'.[133]

It could be argued that Murdock's bestselling book veered towards second-wave feminism rather than the ideals of third-wave feminism and thus its definitions and demarcations of the attributes of masculine and the feminine could be viewed as outdated in the light of subsequent feminist discourse. Her portrayal of gender characteristics was often stereotypical and culturally biased with little account of other cultures' gender

128  Murdock, *The Heroine's Journey*, 85.
129  Ibid., 88.
130  Gloria Durà-Vilà, who lectures at University College London, has differentiated between salutary depression, in other words a dark night, and pathological depression: G. Durà-Vilà et al., 'The Dark Night of the Soul: Causes and Resolution of Emotional Distress among Contemplative Nuns', *Transcultural Psychiatry* 47, no. 4 (1 September 2010): 548–70, <https://doi.org/10.1177/1363461510374899>.
131  Murdock, *The Heroine's Journey*, 90.
132  Ibid., 160.
133  Ibid., 168.

characterisation. Murdock's *The Heroine's Journey* portrays weak mothers from whom the daughter wants to disassociate. However, many daughters who grew up in the west of Ireland in the 1950s and 1960s, for example, experienced a strong matriarchal heritage. While fathers worked in England to provide the family income, mothers who stayed behind not only raised the children, but also ran the farm and took care of the elders. It is not unusual to hear families referred to for generations to the present day as the *Róises*, or the *Pheggies*, a hybrid of the English and Gaelic languages translated as the clan of Rose, or the clan of Peggy. Murdock's book nevertheless constituted a significant intervention in response to Campbell's seminal work and succeeded in marking the descent to the Goddess a crucial element of the awakening journey.

# CHAPTER 5

# Spiritual Awakening: The Women's Voices

## Transformation: Illness as a Creative Process

Abraham Maslow, a key thinker who set the stage for the development of transpersonal theory, argued that creativity and self-actualisation are synonymous: 'My feeling is that the concept of creativeness and the concept of the healthy, self-actualizing, fully human person seem to be coming closer and closer together, and may perhaps turn out to be the same thing'.[1] According to Maslow, the self-actualising process is the process of creativity. All human beings are in the process of creating themselves. This line of thought has precursors. The Danish existentialist philosopher Søren Kierkegaard posited that we create ourselves through our choices, and that it is through our choices we become the persons we are.[2,3] Similarly, Roberto Assagioli developed his theory of psychosynthesis to provide the mechanism of 'the awakening and manifestation of latent potentialities of the human being'.[4] The term awakening, he explained, 'suggests the perception, the becoming aware of a new area of experience, the opening of hitherto closed eyes to an inner reality previously ignored'.[5]

Aspects of spiritual awakening as an outcome of illness featured as a theme in all of the narratives. Its many identifying features included

---

1    A. Maslow, *The Farther Reaches of Human Nature* (New York; Viking Press, 1971), 55.
2    M. Velasquez, *Philosophy: A Text With Readings* (Boston, MA: Cengage Learning, 2010), 180.
3    Søren Kierkegaard, *Either/Or: A Fragment of Life*, trans. L. Swenson and D. Swenson (Princeton, NJ: Princeton University Press, 1949), 141.
4    Assagioli, *Psychosynthesis: A Manual of Principles and Techniques*, 38.
5    Ibid., 40.

transformation, caring for others more as a result of illness, turning points or stimuli for growth and new beginnings, friendship and illness, the mediation of the divine in the world and wisdom gained in illness. Other themes which arose included: prayer; help from beyond the grave; saints; unhealthy understanding of God being healed; people's minds being too small to understand God; following one's intuition, and, finally, gratitude. The latter cluster is not being examined here because the themes did not appear in the majority of the interviews. A decision was made to treat only those themes that were pertinent to the majority.

## Transformation

For the purposes of this research, transformation is defined as a shift from a former way of being to a new way of being which is considered by that person to be more virtuous. In this study, which holds Assagioli's psychosynthesis as a theoretical foundation, transformation implies the integration into everyday life of aspects of the higher unconscious, a latent aspect of human nature in which the 'higher' values or qualities reside, for example: peace, joy, wisdom, compassion and love.

Each of the nine women in the study expressed in various ways, in different language, positive changes in their nature and actions as a result of illness. Identifying features of this theme included: metamorphosis; becoming more one's true self; losing inhibitions; becoming more compassionate towards self and others; discovering a new sense of being looked after by a higher power; seeing the divine in nature and in music; finding the light of God within; discovering a new way of communicating with the divine, and finding one's true gifts and calling.

Angela's expression of finding the light within encapsulated the essence of the theme of transformation:

> there is a presence inside of all of us which is a presence of God I think, it's in there in every single one of us just by virtue of being human, it's in there, but for 99.9%

of us I think it's just covered over, and we can't access it, and there is something about the experience ... through illness which offers you the chance to excavate that capacity within yourself because nothing else is going to save you, nothing else is going to save you ... everybody feels disempowered because they haven't access to that ... that dynamo inside.

Mary Rose now has an informal role as telephone counsellor and is asked to pray for others who are sick. She pondered: 'Maybe our roles change and maybe we are not as aware of what our talents are, we are not aware of what the best path in life is for us ... it's like we want the straight path but sometimes it's the meandering path that brings us to a better destination.' Another type of intelligence emerged for her: 'With illness you have to come up with creative solutions. You end up developing your powers of lateral thinking because you cannot do things the usual tried and tested ways. You have to get a lot more ingenious you have to delve more into yourself and you have to kind of find unique solutions for your situation.'

Sally conveyed the transformation she underwent in a sculpture entitled *Metamorphosis*, which depicted a female figure with roots growing deep into the earth: 'You become much more aware of everything, like I have become aware I can sit outside and watch a spider build a web. I am aware most people have no time to be aware ... you are also more aware of your body ... you evaluate stuff more than I think people who work 9 to 5.' She began to take writing seriously and came to terms with her lesbian orientation, 'I grew more into who I am rather than what people decided I should be, because I think I always lived to what other people thought was good for me.'

Angela found her voice as a singer of sacred chant during her illness and said that her invisible illness presented her with an opportunity for growth: 'When you look at the world ... and you look at people you know being driven by material needs and being you know incapable of managing their emotions ... there is an opportunity to learn an alternative way of being that is given sometime.' She now wants to put what she has learned to good use, 'I want to apply what I have learned both in singing and in ritual chant and in meditation and in illness, somewhere. And the idea is to make a tool that I would investigate what need is met by applying ritual chant and song in palliative care.'

Alice's chemical sensitivity makes it difficult for her to go to church services and she has discovered a new sense of the divine in other ways, 'Because I couldn't go to churches, I found out in the countryside I never felt alone, just to look up at the sky and look around.' She also devotes time to praying for her family and feels that her prayer has saved one of her nieces who had been involved in a road accident overseas. Patricia found that she developed a greater sense of what matters during her illness. She explored Buddhist meditation and mindfulness for her pain and found that this helped her to let go of anxiety around teachings on hell with which she had been indoctrinated: 'The more I would get into things like that (meditation) the more the other seems, you know the way I am split, half of me thinks I am going to hell you know deep down, not in my logical rational self but you know my subconscious, and then the other part thinks, "no, that's crazy."'

Retired nurse Julia's attitude to her own nursing profession and to medicine changed as a consequence of her illness and not being believed by doctors. She began to visit complementary therapists and healers and developed an interest in a more holistic paradigm of medicine: 'I could see another whole different world, the natural world that we had all forgotten about, and that's the way I have gone since then.' She began to experience paranormal encounters, visions and mystical experiences. A near-death experience pointed her to a new vocation as an environmental campaigner: 'Maybe this is my work, to get it out, to get electro-sensitivity out there, get it known.'

Rachel learned to take care of herself better as a result of illness. In addition, she reported increased empathy with suffering others. She now corresponds with a number of prisoners and supplies them with books. Sharon's was the marginal voice proclaiming that the illness had nothing good about it, in contrast to the other interviewees who were enthusiastic to talk about their growth in adversity. Notwithstanding this negative position on her illness, she related a change of attitude around suicide, 'I used to think that we all had the right to take our lives if we considered that the life we were living wasn't worth it.' She also spoke about having a new feeling, since becoming ill, that she is being looked after by a higher power, 'I do have the sense that I am being looked after even though it sounds really bizarre to say it, because if I was being looked after why did I get sick? It's like I have been looked after somehow since getting sick. I don't know what it is, whether it's spirit guides or whatever, I would have a bit of a sense of that before, but since getting sick I know it for sure. I haven't been allowed to die.'

In the above accounts what is clearly evident is that each participant spontaneously identified a change in their perspective or participation in the flow of life. They have identified within themselves an evolution of personality which was unexpected. The illness had drawn the person into excavating their own inner resources and, in undertaking this task, certain historical rigidities fell away and a new dimension of personhood came into view. Transformation was tangible and practical in each life narrative.

In a parallel process, my own story featured themes of transformation through illness including gains of deeper states of wisdom and awareness, and a revolution from feeling powerless in illness to becoming an academic researcher on the topic of inner growth in invisible illness.

## Stimuli for Transformation and Spiritual Awakening

This section aims to discern a further feature of the spiritual awakening process, namely the catalysing forces for the turning points which enabled spiritual awakening, transformation or a deepening in wisdom for the participants. It endeavours to name specific characteristics of the illness experience which may have offered the opportunity for a shift from anguish to wisdom.

For Mary Rose, for example, the catalyst for awakening was the isolating effect of illness – isolation brought the solitude which enabled her to tune into her deepest wisdom. In this excerpt from her narrative, she refers to a passage in the book *Eat, Pray, Love*. She compared and contrasted the experience of a person who is ill to that of the author of the book, Elizabeth

Gilbert.[6] Mary Rose selected relevant passages from the book which is a memoir of the author's spiritual quest:

> The search for God is a reversal of the normal mundane order, according to *Eat, Pray Love*, and in our illness the normal mundane order is removed from us and maybe we end up finding God as a consequence. Quoting Gilbert: 'In search for God you revert from what attracts you and swim toward that which is difficult.' Now that's in the search for God, that's a conscious choice, but for us we haven't any choice, and we often can't follow what attracts us and we feel forced into the flow of what is difficult, we didn't choose to swim towards it – well I didn't anyway – but you're kind of forced into a different slipstream. And maybe we are doing things that we wouldn't have done and maybe we end up growing in ways we wouldn't have grown if we hadn't been forced out of the norm, forced out of our norm.

Here, I attempt to harvest catalysts for awakening from the narratives of the other women who took part in this study. Similar to Mary Rose's case, Angela proffered that the isolation concomitant with her illness was what enabled her to grow:

> It's an enforced period of withdrawal, in many ways it's a huge opportunity, it's very hard to see it as an opportunity when you are in it and it's very hard to see that you are actually quite privileged to be given that I think. But that's actually what it is, I mean when you look at the state of the world ... there is an opportunity you know to learn an alternative way of being that is given sometimes, and you have to have the ears to hear it, that there is some kind of privilege in it – there is some sense of the hand of God in it.

An encounter with Sahaj Marg meditation represented Angela's turning point, she has now practised it for twenty years: 'You have to learn devotion to your own heart, because nobody else believes in you, everybody else just thinks you are for the birds. You have to learn compassion, devotion and you have to learn where the love really is, it's inside yourself and it's the only thing that we all want.'

Alice, after her misdiagnosis as anorexic had been acknowledged by doctors, had a near-death experience whilst in hospital undergoing an

6    E. Bailey Gilbert, *Eat, Pray, Love: One Woman's Search for Everything Across Italy, India and Indonesia* (Princeton, NJ: Penguin Books, 2007), 184.

operation related to her bowel. After that she felt that she was being taken care of by forces from another dimension: 'I remember having this beautiful yellow light, absolutely gorgeous light and in that light was my grandmother and an uncle-in-law that had died. It was absolutely peaceful and then I heard the doctors say: "Look! We have her back! We have her back! We have a pulse!"'

Sally advises anyone who is chronically ill to look at their most inner being, indicating that she had done the same, 'To look at your most inner being and to look at the world immediately around you and don't look for miracles, because they are not there, don't look for a doctor somewhere else to fix you because it is you who knows what you need ... I think the holy Grail is inside ourselves and we can find a way to live with this illness well.'

Though Sharon at the time of the interview expressed that her life had been ruined, it was clear from her narrative that there had been a turning point towards a new will to live when she found acceptance from other people who were ill or had experienced major trauma. Their kindness kept her alive, she said:

> I have gained friendship with the most amazing people and I consider myself very blessed. So yeah, I mourn the friendships that I have lost. There are other friends who do understand, but most of them it's because they've been through something pretty traumatic in their lives themselves and I mean they are just fantastic. It's just that they are just pure compassion, and that's the only word I can think of, and empathy, and yeah, it's like a meeting of the souls.

Orla was pleased that a doctor had advised her that she had to learn how to manage her illness herself:

> People are always looking for an answer, but the way of coping is not to find an answer, the way of coping I think is to say okay, this is the hand I have been dealt, this is the situation. Every time you go through a crisis like that, just in my life it just happens to be illness, you find a mechanism that's going to slot right in, I did that.

Patricia had self-medicated with alcohol for some years to numb the physical pain and became addicted. For her, the twelve-step programme of AA presented a turning point, she credited the spiritual teaching of AA for enabling her to jettison, to some degree, the fear of hell with which she had been raised. 'I think building up that other belief in a higher power which would be different. My idea of a higher power is all the good that's out there.'

Julia's turning point towards a deeper level of spirituality constituted the stream of mystical experiences she began to have following her sense of despair about being let down by her own profession, the medical world: 'I was dead really to what I knew, and a whole lot of all these strange things then started happening.' These strange things included hearing benign voices, out-of-body experiences, feeling guided to sacred places, and a sense of close communion with saints and angels. These experiences led to her gaining a whole new understanding of spirituality which in turn gifted her with empowerment and a refusal to have her electro-sensitivity dismissed by doctors and officials.

The above account shows that participants could mark with ease the turning points in their illness after which they began to experience spiritual awakening. Catalysing forces for growth are evident in these narratives. Transformation was attributed to the enforced isolation in which illness bears characteristics of a meditation. Looking at the inner life as opposed to expecting a cure from outside, meeting people with similar illnesses, mystical experiences as well as empowering advice from a doctor all had powerful transformative effects on meaning-making in the course of illness.

Principal catalysing forces for change in my personal narrative bear resonance to the above accounts. A major theme of my story featured the way in which visits to holistic therapists, including an astrologer, resulted in an expanded spiritual horizon. I referred also to a particular book on spiritual healing which was to become a catalytic agent in my spiritual awakening:

> I was still in a state of shock and awakening of a new consciousness as I travelled on the train, like I had just heard news that was terribly serious and had massive implications for my life ... it was a definite turning point in my life ... the missing link, the 'aha' moment.

Visits to practitioners which are at various times referred to as alternative, holistic, esoteric, shamanistic, complementary, metaphysical or 'New Age' constitute a major theme in my personal narrative. In particular, there is a focus in the narrative on spiritual awakening occurring as a result of such practices. For the purposes of this theme, the definition of holistic delineated by Robert Fuller, Professor of Religion at Bradley University, Illinois, provides a useful understanding of the worldview underpinning holistic practices. According to Fuller, in the holistic paradigm the world is viewed 'not as the aggregate of separate material parts but rather as the living expression of an underlying spiritual energy (God).'[7] In a chapter concerning holistic health practices in *Spirituality and the Secular Quest* (1996), a book from a projected twenty-five-volume encyclopaedia on world spiritualities, Fuller further elucidated the world view of holistic therapies:

> The body, because it belongs to the more expansive cosmos, is said to have inner access to the creative powers by which life itself is possible. Alternative healing techniques are predicated upon the belief that under certain conditions extra-mundane forces enter into, and exert sanative influences upon, the human realm. They are therefore substantively spiritual. They seek to induce consciousness of a sudden, felt intrusion of a 'More' that is experienced as other than the material world and thereafter replaces all other forms of reality as normative or ultimately meaningful.[8]

In my story, spiritual awakening wasn't consciously pursued. It happened as a result of a search for help with health and confidence issues. During my twenties in London, there was a gap between my level of self-confidence on the one hand, and a desire to be successful in the world, on the other. I attribute my initiation into spirituality to the frustration resulting from this struggle to succeed, and also to low energy and frequent debilitating chest infections. During the first year in London I began to consult an astrologer in an effort to find some solutions and this led to what I now see as an enlightenment of my consciousness as this quote from the narrative illustrates:

> My spiritual awakening happened through searching for help with my life. I discovered astrology. That woke me up to new possibilities. My astrologer became a soul friend ... I was opened up to the healing power of listening, of being seen and respected by another human being.

---

7    R. Fuller, 'Holistic Health Practices', in *Spirituality and the Secular Quest*, ed. P. van Ness (New York: The Crossroad Publishing Company, 1996), 230.
8    Ibid.

The choice of consulting an astrologer as opposed to seeking help from institutional religion may be contextualised by research undertaken by dialogue partners Paul Heelas and Linda Woodhead from Lancaster University. The latter researchers chose the town of Kendal in Cumbria, with a population of 28,000, as a base to investigate whether holistic therapies were replacing Christianity in Britain.[9] Their conclusions were published in 2004 in *The Spiritual Revolution: Why Religion is Giving Way to Spirituality*.[10] The scholars carried out a church attendance count and found that 7.9 per cent of the population attended church services. Their survey of the holistic milieu showed that 1.6 per cent took part in activities of the 'new spirituality'. The research conducted established that the new spirituality had grown by 300 per cent during the 1990s. Heelas and Woodhead concluded that, 'If the holistic milieu continues to grow at the same linear rate that it has since 1970 and if the congregational domain continues to decline at the same rate that it has during the same period, then the spiritual revolution would take place during the third decade of the third millennium'.[11]

Robert Fuller, a sociologist of religion, has offered useful insights into the topic of holistic healing practices and their benefits for spiritual awakening. In the USA, Fuller found high educational standards amongst advocates of holistic practices, 'Most of those attracted to holistic forms of healing are self-styled progressive thinkers and find scriptural religion intellectually obsolete. Their curiosity about exploring the connections between the physical and metaphysical dimensions of the universe runs too far afield from the conceptual constraints of Jewish or Christian theology'.[12]

Fuller asserted that holistic healing acts as a carrier of spiritual awakening and compares them, in their transformational abilities, to the initiation rites of ancient religions: 'Holistic healing practices evoke a sense of wonder

---

9    <http://www.lancaster.ac.uk/fss/projects/ieppp/kendal/>. Accessed 11 May 2015.
10   P. Heelas et al., *The Spiritual Revolution: Why Religion Is Giving Way to Spirituality*, 1st edn (Chichester: Wiley-Blackwell, 2004).
11   Ibid., 45.
12   Fuller, 'Holistic Health Practices', 244.

and mystery that supplies an experiential context for believing that one has discovered the primal reality on which life is ultimately dependent'.[13]

Fuller argued that there was a similarity of transformation experienced by newcomers to holistic healing systems, proffering that they 'go through cognitive and experiential transformations' very similar to those people taking the initiation ceremony in traditional initiation rites in archaic religions.[14] He was referring to the scholarship of religious anthropologist Mircea Eliade (1907–1986), who had studied patterns in initiation ceremonies in tribal cultures. Eliade explored how those societies created rituals in which old structures of the personality could be dissolved or enabled to undergo a 'death', in order to make way for a deeper level of consciousness to emerge.[15]

## Wisdom Gained from Illness

Wisdom gained as a result of illness featured as a motif in all of the narratives. The identifying features of this theme included the notion that people with invisible illnesses are barometers for the future of the world, empowerment, training of doctors, the afterlife, life is not meant to be easy, the effect of electro-magnetic rays on people, love does not have to be merited, and life's choices.

Mary Rose believes that people with illnesses like hers could be seen as laboratory evidence of the damage being done to all human beings by chemicals and electro-magnetic radiation:

13　Ibid., 246.
14　R. Fuller, 'Subtle Energies and the American Metaphysical Tradition', in *Religion and Healing in America* (Oxford: Oxford University Press, 2005), 383.
15　M. Eliade, *Rites and Symbols of Initiation*, 1st edn (Dallas, TX; New York: Spring, 1998).

There's a term 'the canary in the mine'. The canaries were sent down the mine to check if the air was good enough for the miners to go down so some people, like the canaries in the mine, they are like the litmus paper for what societies do in general. But the effects of society and how it lives in general, some people are more sensitive to the effects than others. The effects of even the use of chemicals I mean people don't understand sometimes that one chemical might be okay but if you have a plug-in [air freshener] in your house, and you have a lot of sprays, and you use a lot of cleaning substances – the combination of them all might be too much for your immune system; but because people have become used to all these things in society they don't analyse their effects. People like me tend to show up the effects of so-called progress more than others; and some things that in 20 years' time they might discover were harmful, we already discovered they are harmful, but the long-term studies might not be done for another 20 years.

On radiation pollution matters, Julia tries to generate awareness about the effects of radiation and electro-sensitivity: 'Just the electricity was killing us all in one way or another you know, well it was our own mast really that radiated the microwaves, we are all being microwaved out of it.' She began to take a fresh look at her former profession of medicine as a result of her health crisis, 'I was looking at what they were doing, and I said they are killing everybody with tablets.' Her illness led her to perceive wisdom in complementary healing practices, 'I could see another whole different world, the natural world that we had all forgotten about.'

Angela's growth in wisdom is oriented inwards. She claims that people are by and large disempowered in the world, driven by material needs and feeling unhappy because they are not in touch with their inner light: 'We are so lost, we are seeing a reflection of disempowerment in each other all the time, everybody feels disempowered, because they haven't access to that, that thing that, that dynamo inside, that light.' Alice's narrative highlighted a potential for improvement in the training of doctors because of the negative consequences she suffered as a result of doctors equating her physical illness with anorexia: 'All the doctors I met, none of them would listen to me, they all kind of went their own way, but I can't blame any of them because that's the way they are trained ... I have to look at it that way because none of them were cruel, they just missed things they just didn't, they didn't do their job properly.'

For Sharon, the deep connection which she called 'a pool of love' with people who suffer from invisible illnesses, gave her some idea of what life after death might look like: 'All I can think of is it's just this pool of love that we came from and that one day we'll go back to, and I think people who have experienced something like a lot of us have, and that's the only thing I am grateful for in this illness.'

These accounts indicate that the participants unearthed deep wisdom during their illness in a spectrum of areas. Wisdom is evident in the metaphor of 'the canaries down the mine' – the damage caused by chemicals to people who have multiple chemical sensitivity could be seen as a warning for the future of society. Astute observations – that people are suffering from disempowerment because they have no access to their inner light, that life is not meant to be smooth, that nature can bring healing, that drugs are being over prescribed, that people don't have to earn divine love, that suffering in illness can lead to a pool of love, and that doctors are not to blame but their training needs to be modified – all display wisdom, good judgement and forgiveness gained as a consequence of illness. Materialism, greed and the fast pace of life are understood as disempowering for human beings.

## The Mediation of the Divine in the World

The way the divine is heard or the manner in which it makes itself known is the essence of this theme which emerged in seven of the nine interviews. It had varying identifying features and illustrates an emerging relationship in how the divine is perceived and attended to.

Features of this theme included listening to the God within, new ways of discerning how to go forward in life, a life-altering encounter with a meditation practice, divine qualities being transmitted through music and nature, synchronicity, and mystical experiences. The motif is eloquently epitomised in this statement by Mary Rose:

> I have found since I got sick that I have become more open to the God within and
> I would tune into the God within us ... I have become a lot more open to that, that
> God is within us as well, and I wasn't really tuned into that bit of it at all until I got
> sick. When you're sick you're inclined to listen to what's within.

Mary Rose described illness as a time when all the signposts disappear, but this leads to a new way of discernment: 'You can get too used to just navigating by the same signposts the whole time and sometimes when the signposts are taken away it makes you look for a new ones.' She also spoke of experiencing the presence of Archangel Raphael in a session with a spiritual healer, and has had other mystical experiences which gifted a sense of comfort. Angela received a connection to pure love through her Sahaj Marg meditation practice, 'I got that connection to pure love for the first time I think in my experience on this planet.' Alice's chemical sensitivity changed the location of communion with the divine for her. She no longer could attend church as she cannot be near perfumes, after-shave products and other chemical residue. She now listens to sacred music on a classical radio station on Sunday mornings, saying that this is now her Mass. She spoke also of finding spirituality in nature. Sharon has a new sense of a higher power looking after her.

Orla has struggled with illness on and off since childhood which makes it difficult to detect which changes came about as a result of illness itself. Though raised a strict Catholic, her religion is more eclectic now. She spoke about being attentive to the window that illness opens up when the door on good health has been shut, 'if you keep your mind and heart and eyes open for the window that's going to open, your life can change in amazing ways.' Julia's multiple metaphysical experiences led her to feel she was getting direction from dreams, from saints and from angels. This radical shift in her spiritual life enabled her to be more empowered in life. Rachel described a vision of an ethereal light as she sat in her sitting room. This experience profoundly affected her life and put her mind to rest in relation to a quest for truth about the nature of God: 'I couldn't describe how beautiful it was, it was so beautiful, and it was so loving, so loving. I remember I just gaped and gaped, I remember I kept on saying in my mind something like: "Stay! I want to stay with you." And it lasted long enough to really know it was happening.'

This account illustrates distinctive shifts in how the divine is perceived and mediated in the world. Illness provided opportunities to abandon images of God as external in favour of an internal experience, to perceive God as love, to experience the divine in nature, to feel that there is a benevolent higher power in charge of life. Mystical experiences led to a perception of God as a loving entity. A sense of empowerment and inner peace resulting from changes in beliefs about the nature of the divine is evident in these accounts where participants speak of feeling loved and cared for by a divine source. A sense of composure and gentle self-confidence is communicated in these accounts of individual experiences of the nature of the divine.

We see that the women managed to throw off the shackles of their spiritual conditioning and 'grow up', to use the expression of Ken Wilber, on their spiritual trajectory. Borrowing here from Jean Gebser (1905–1973), Wilber delineated seven stages of development that human consciousness progresses through in all 'lines' of intelligence. Applying Wilber's ideas, the new inner freedom expressed by the women, their care for the cosmos, openness to diverse forms of spiritual practice, and expanded worldview denotes a progression from the mythic level or stage of consciousness to a pluralistic one. The problem with the magic and mythic literal levels of spiritual intelligence, according to Wilber, is that they are at a low level of spiritual intelligence, and yet they are the most common worldwide. Most of the major world religions are stuck at the magic and mythic level, even though the higher levels are available in each religion.[16]

The women's narratives concur with my own experience of a shift in how the divine is experienced. My story recalls an expression of Catholicism in my religious upbringing which had oppressive characteristics. I later dropped out of the Church for many years owing to what I described as being, 'indoctrinated with notions of our personal sinfulness. It told me that I was born with original sin.' A new perception of God emerged in the course of illness: 'A loving God, a God that was more of an energy force permeating me than a judgemental figure in the heavens.'

---

16   K. Wilber, *Integral Spirituality: A Startling New Role for Religion in the Modern and Postmodern World*, reprint edn (Boston, MA: Shambhala, 2007).

As part of my personal quest for healing as well as for research, I have taken part in a body therapy which honours symptoms of illness as bearers of divine energy. This work has enabled me to awaken spiritually through applying deep attention to body symptoms.

Founded by Arnold Mindell, *process oriented* psychotherapy, also known as *process work*, holds that meaning is reached through honouring the felt sense of the symptoms. Instead of seeing symptoms and disturbances as pathologies to be healed or transcended, process oriented psychology considers them to be crucial expressions of what we need for our further growth and development. Mindell has stated:

> Whether fate is called acute or chronic illness, academic or business failure, sexual hang-up, insanity, suicide, or secret love affair, the pattern for living the dreaming-body hovers in the background as the antidote to pain. Our biggest problems seem to be meant to interrupt life and awaken us to our total capacity, warriorship, and death, to end our earlier personality and find the path of heart.[17]

In his classic work *Dreambody: The Body's Role in Revealing the Self* (1998), Arnold Mindell claims that symptoms are self-healing: 'Symptoms are their own healers; when you begin to work on them, they are self-curing in the sense of self-revealing'.[18] In the process oriented approach, body sensations, the felt sense of symptoms, dreams, altered states, and relationship troubles are all worked with in order to develop greater awareness, understanding and compassion.

Mindell contends that most of us live in what he terms *consensus reality*, the reality of every life, working, shopping, socialising, without going deeper: 'Consensus and social rules seem to repress signs from the unconscious. The reality most people follow seems to forbid you from investigating your hallucinations, aches and pains, and accidents'.[19] In process theory, my curiosity about my trance like states and subjective experiences of illness are construed as *secondary attention* which is a different form of

---

17    A. Mindell, *The Shaman's Body: A New Shamanism for Transforming Health, Relationships, and Community* (San Francisco, CA: HarperSanFrancisco, 1993), 15.
18    Mindell, *Dreambody: The Body's Role in Revealing the Self*, 22.
19    Mindell, *The Shaman's Body*, 9.

consciousness to everyday consciousness. *Primary attention* refers to our normal consciousness and consensus reality. *Secondary attention* attends to another level of reality which he calls the *dreambody*, and is expressed in dreams, bodily sensations and symptoms. It is often only in states of illness that we give any attention to secondary reality: 'Your ego does not die easily, and so you listen to subtle feelings and sensations only when they threaten to kill you'.[20]

Mindell posits that body sensations are similar to dreams. Process oriented therapy treats symptoms and sensations in a similar way to working with dreams: 'If you say that you are tired, or have a sore throat, for example, you are reporting on momentary body or proprioceptive feelings. Although these feelings may begin as fatigue or a sore throat, if you get closer to and into them – if you consciously immerse yourself and climb into them – they soon flow on and evolve as a dreaming process'.[21]

The following is a journal extract written after a process oriented psychotherapy session which specifically focused on my ME symptoms. This brief description of a process work session illustrates how symptoms, if they are experienced in a phenomenological manner, can have a wise message and bring the person who is suffering to a place of peace with a sense of meaning and enlightenment. Bríd, to whom I refer in the extract, is the therapist.

> Today I worked on the ME/Lyme symptoms. I had been feeling tired. I sat in the chair and described the symptoms, what it was like in my body. Exhaustion, sore throat, itchy eyes, etc. I slumped in the chair, arms hanging down. I said it was like a cloud. Then I said it was like being dead, but there were things like wire scrubbers in my head with electricity going through them. There were itches and my clothes were annoying me. She asked me to go deeper into the experience. I felt like a floppy thing. It was saying 'leave me alone I don't want to do anything.' Then I had the urge to go forward flopped over my knees. Eventually I lay down on the ground. Bríd half mimics what I do, in support. When I am on the ground she is on the ground trying to feel into my experience. I lay on the floor stretched out, my head lying on my outstretched arm.

20   Ibid., 10.
21   Ibid., 21.

I felt into this. I said it felt really good, the energy shifted and I felt glad in my heart
to have permission to feel into Floppy and be seen in it by another. So happy to
relax and do nothing.
This all took ages with few words being spoken.
Then I felt that I wanted to mould into the earth, to be sucked in by the earth. I saw
coffins in the earth and wanted to be one of the bodies, totally at peace and at one
with the earth. She encouraged me to feel deeply into it. I felt part of the earth, the
soil. Flowers grew out of me but I did nothing. Climates and winds and seas happened but I was still.
She asked me to feel into the spirit of the earth. I said I felt generous, at peace, just
being, totally accepting of everything that came into me, bodies and all.
Totally accepting of all that goes on. Totally happy.
Bríd then asked me what did I think of the other Bernadette who was busy and
wanted to be busy. I said she needed me with her in order to be grounded, but that
she didn't trust me. I wanted to take her into my heart.
Eventually the session was nearly over so I slowly stood up, and merged the two balls
of energy, Bernadette who wants to do, and Bernadette who is part of the earth and
is happy and accepting of everything. I held one in both hands, stretched out, and
brought the two together.

The session ended with feelings of peace. Although not a 'cure' in the
orthodox sense, Mindell postulated that deeper healing and wholeness
can be facilitated by process work: 'According to medicine people living in
native settings around the world, and to mystical traditions, the shaman's
dreamingbody, when accessed, is a source of health, personal growth, good
relationships, and a sense of community'.[22]

22    Ibid., 3.

# CHAPTER 6

# Key Themes Arising from the Research as a Whole

Six overarching themes emerged from this exploratory study as a whole, from the consideration of the literature from medical humanities, through to a select review of theories of spiritual awakening, and finally to the analysis of the women's narratives.

1.  Testimonial injustice and spiritual awakening: the most traumatising aspect of the illness for the women participants was not being believed. Yet it was this deepest hurt that catalysed their spiritual awakening.
2.  Invisible illness, patriarchal medicine and the patriarchal God: this thread concerns the way in which the patriarchal feature of medical practice corresponds to a pervasiveness of patriarchal images and ideas of God in Western culture.
3.  Narrative as a facilitator of spiritual awakening: having one's testimony heard may bring a powerful transformational outcome.
4.  Spirit speaks through illness: a call for a new medical paradigm.
5.  Illness as portal to creativity and wisdom: the opportunities inherent in illness.
6.  Illness, solitude and spiritual awakening: solitude as a fundamental constituent on the path of spiritual awakening.

This chapter reflects on these key insights.

## Testimonial Injustice and Spiritual Awakening

We have seen that living with invisible illness and the precipitation of spiritual awakening are deeply intertwined in the narratives of the women who were at the heart of this research. The preceding discussion hints at some of the dynamics which are at work in this interconnection. The first dynamic is the profound experience of injustice through which many people living with invisible illness pass. It is a fact of history that many great mystics have emerged from deep immersion in the experience of injustice and so it is too in the field of illness.

Philosopher Havi Carel, has argued that people who are ill are vulnerable to *epistemic injustice*. Here she is referring to the theories of Miranda Fricker, a philosopher at the University of Sheffield, who has published an insightful book entitled *Epistemic Injustice: Power and the Ethics of Knowing* (2007). Fricker has delineated two forms of epistemic injustice, each of which is driven by a form of prejudice: *testimonial* injustice and *hermeneutical* injustice. Testimonial injustice arises in prejudices which accord a 'deflated level of credibility to a speaker's word'.[1] This is a class of injustice in which someone is 'wronged specifically in her capacity as a knower'.[2] Hermeneutical injustice pertains to the type of inequality experienced by people who have no access to resources, for instance, the appropriate kind of education, which would help them make sense of their experiences. Those who experience this kind of injustice may, as a consequence, be less likely to believe their own testimonies.

Sustained by Fricker's arguments, Carel proposes that people who are chronically ill are vulnerable to testimonial injustice 'through the presumptive attribution of characteristics like cognitive unreliability and emotional instability that downgrade the credibility of their testimonies'.[3] She further

---

1    M. Fricker, *Epistemic Injustice: Power and the Ethics of Knowing* (Oxford; New York: Oxford University Press, 2007), 1.
2    Ibid., 20.
3    H. Carel and I. Kidd, 'Epistemic Injustice in Healthcare: A Philosophical Analysis', *Medicine, Health Care, and Philosophy* 17, no. 4 (November 2014): 529, <https://doi.org/10.1007/s11019-014-9560-2>.

argues that epistemic injustice occurs because of the existence of its converse position, *epistemic privilege* which is afforded to medical doctors because of their training, allowing them to maintain 'certain styles of articulating ... in ways that marginalise ill persons'.[4]

Throughout this research project, the deep experience of injustice which haunts the experience of invisible illness has been highlighted. It suggests that the roots of the experience of some illnesses being discredited by the medical profession may be traced to the Flexner Report in 1910. Though this report resulted in vast improvements in medical training, it also yielded the negative consequence of an over-emphasis on rigid scientific methodologies in medicine and relegated soft skills such as empathy with the suffering patient to a lesser position. By way of challenge in 1969, the seeds of a medical humanities movement were sown, when academics and physicians including the founder of medical ethics, Edmund Pellegrino, convened to address how the *wounded humanity* of the patient could be embraced by medicine. Both Arthur Kleinman, medical anthropologist and humanitarian, and Rita Charon, the founder of *narrative medicine*, have taken up the campaign for the lived experience of the patient to be fittingly recognised primarily by means of attentive listening to the patient – in other words acting as agents of testimonial justice. As in any contestation of practical expressions of justice, both Kleinman and Charon acknowledged frequent conflicts between what the established powers (doctor) sees as the cause of the disease, and the (advocate) patient's testimony.

The experience of testimonial injustice was intensified for the interview participants because it was often entwined with a perennial, religion-based, gender struggle which has sought to overcome the unrelenting lack of validation of women's testimony. We have noted that Maria Harris is an iconic figure for women's spiritual freedom as she has urged them to become aware of internalised untruths from society's accounts of the Judeo-Christian tradition about their lack of religious power and authority; Harris has illustrated how women who come to recognise the lack of truth in these internalised beliefs will spiritually awaken. Similarly, Beverly

4    Ibid.

Lanzetta maintained that suppression of women in the spheres of religion and society constitutes violence against their embodiment of the divine in the world and affects their health. She proposed a path towards awakening and empowerment based on the journey of Teresa of Avila, who overcame prejudice directed against her because of her gender. In a manner akin to the journey of the women described in this research, Teresa did this by feeling her gender-grounded wounds at a deep level which thus enabled the birth of her full humanity in deeply creative and innovative interventions which are being appropriated with even greater energy as time passes. Indeed, the renowned French feminist linguist and psychoanalyst Julia Kristeva believes that Teresa of Avila 500 years ago revealed to her readers a new kind of feminine insight that the body is deeply conversant with the soul.

As in Teresa's narrative, a perpetual traumatising experience which had failed to be acknowledged was the bedrock of the participants' spiritual awakening. Trauma emerged as an overarching theme in the results of the study and although some aspects of the trauma were caused by the illness itself, the overarching source of trauma was the lack of belief by the medical profession. Testimonial injustice was clearly evident in the descriptions of how the women had not been believed by doctors because their test results were negative. It was clear that a prejudice abides by which the word of the woman with invisible illness is not given credibility and she is 'wronged specifically in her capacity as a knower'.[5]

Trauma related to testimonial injustice snowballed as the women experienced a falling away of friends and associates who did not believe in the reality of the illness because of the initial disbelieving response of the medical profession. Subsequently, because doctors could find no physical disease in their tests, participants suffered further testimonial injustice, trauma and stigma by having their physical illness equated to a mental illness. Hurtful comments uttered by the medical profession as well as by family, friends and associates came as a direct consequence of the failure of medical tests to show up a physical disease and ultimately gave way to disbelief. Disbelief had the further knock-on consequences of isolation,

5    Fricker, *Epistemic Injustice*, 20.

intensified marginalisation, and absence of the kind of support ordinarily expected in times of illness.

While justice and mysticism are often brought into dialogue in the context of activist spiritualities of protest and liberation, what is unique in this study is the discovery that it is a form of injustice (testimonial) and its traumatic wounding of those who are affected that is the key to the spiritual awakening of those who participated in this study.

It is interesting to note that Robert Grant's psycho-spiritual approach to trauma contributes a framework which illuminates spiritual awakening through the experience of chronic invisible illnesses arising from its inherent traumas. He contended that trauma is often necessary for spiritual awakening today: 'In the current Zeitgeist (spirit of the times) the ego is the only reality most victims have ever known. Normally it takes the gut-wrenching pain of trauma to expose the ego's limitations'.[6] In his view, the type of marginalisation which is a feature of invisible illness may be an aid to becoming more authentic human beings: 'The path of the marginalised is the path of all trauma victims. It is also the path of liberation and spiritual growth. To be marginal is to be cast out of the "taken for granted" which in many cases is blind, sedated and thus the illusory version of reality'.[7]

## Invisible Illness, Patriarchal Medicine, and the Patriarchal God

The second thread that weaves through the research is the way in which the patriarchal characteristic of medical practice coincides with a prevalence of patriarchal images of God in Western culture. Both features bore a crucial impact on the health and wellbeing of the women who participated in the study. The reductionist scientific model of medicine, in which the doctor tends towards wielding power over the patient mirrors the archetype of

6    Grant, *The Way of the Wound*, 100.
7    Ibid., 34.

a God who is external to the individual, male and authoritarian. Persons can be considered beings-in-relationship, and illness can be considered a disruption in biological relationships that in turn affects all the other relational aspects of a person. Spirituality concerns a person's relationship with transcendence. Therefore, genuinely holistic health care must address the totality of the patient's relational existence: physical, psychological, social and spiritual.

Despite laudable efforts on behalf of advocates of medical humanities who have sought to give power back to the patient, the reductionist medical model is still, in practice, entrenched in cultural attitudes which have been described as 'patriarchal' by Alan Bleakley, Professor of Medical Education and Medical Humanities at Plymouth University Peninsula School of Medicine.[8] Bleakley blames this male bias in medicine on the educational system prevailing in doctors' training:

> The current orthodoxy in curriculum planning, such as behavioural outcomes-based learning – expressed as competencies – can be seen as rational, technical, instrumental, hierarchical, goal-oriented and cold, thus resembling the classic profile of the masculine protest and the authoritarian personality. Such approaches deny process, intuition and affect as legitimate learning.[9]

One of the effects of such a bias in medical training on participants in this study has been a sense of alienation, shaming, and emotional diminishment when their testimony of illness was not believed.

Beverly Lanzetta has linked this type of violence against women to spiritual oppression, such as the oppression Teresa of Avila suffered when her spiritual accounts were decried by her spiritual doctors of the Catholic Church. Lanzetta has argued that women's spiritual oppression is the foundation of all of women's oppression: 'This fundamental belief in women's spiritual inferiority inevitably permeates the cultural imagination, and contributes to and fosters violent acts against women.'[10]

8    A. Bleakley, 'Gender Matters in Medical Education', *Medical Education* 47, no. 1 (January 2013): 66, <https://doi.org/10.1111/j.1365-2923.2012.04351.x>.
9    Ibid., 66–7.
10   Lanzetta, *Radical Wisdom*, 68.

In her book *Radical Wisdom*, Lanzetta has deliberated on:

> a continual and subtle form of violence directed against them [women] that is dif-
> ficult to name. Part of this difficulty has to do with the interior levels on which these
> wounds take place, in which what is most vulnerable and intimate about a person is
> subjected to forms of oppression outside the bounds of accepted social discourse.[11]

Elsewhere Lanzetta has criticised, with particular reference to many wom-
en's experiences in the healthcare system, what she called a 'Cartesian model
of reductionism':

> Corporate forms of oppression are present when the medical community applies a
> model of Cartesian reductionism to the spiritual implications of women's health;
> dismisses or denies gender differences in research, diagnosis, and treatment plans;
> or trivializes women's ailments as symptomatic, psychosomatic, or hysterical.[12]

Lanzetta viewed the core wound suffered by women as the split between
mind and body, and the superior position given to rationality over spirituality. She argued that there exists 'a disturbing tradition in Western spirituality
that forcefully denies women's capacity for becoming divine'.[13] Crucially,
she posited that key to spiritual awakening for women is healing the wound
of the feminine through the mystical path; it is 'through feminist mystical
consciousness that women are healed of the wounds of inequality and sub-
ordination, and find the strength to claim themselves as spiritual authorities in their own right'.[14] Lanzetta named the path to spiritual awakening,
which can enable women to become empowered by healing deep spiritual
wounds, the *via feminina*. Part of the journey consists of confronting 'the
injustice and violence within which the terms *female-feminine-woman* have
been inscribed throughout recorded human history'.[15] It would involve a
radical pulling up the roots of misogyny and seeds of oppression that have
been handed down from generation to generation.

11   Ibid., 9.
12   Lanzetta, 'Women, Soul Wounds, and Integrative Medicine', 91.
13   Lanzetta, *Radical Wisdom*, 11.
14   Ibid., 12.
15   Ibid., 16.

Lanzetta argued that, 'History, philosophy, theology, and literature, as well as legal, social and political codes, were established and written by men. As daughter, wife, and mother, females were the property of males and gender stratification was maintained through complex economic arrangements, power disparities, and social controls endorsed by Church and state'.[16] Lanzetta's *via feminina* would seek to heal the wound at the core of womanhood. As a path to spiritual awakening, the via feminina pays particular attention to integrating and incorporating the multiple wisdoms of body, psyche and soul in order to name and heal what offends, diminishes, or violates women. This is a path to liberate women from 'what diminishes, injures, humiliates or shames her – to a positive affirmation of her dignity and worth'.[17]

Lanzetta termed this kind of post-modern quest for healing and liberation *contemplative* or *mystical* feminism. This journey of spiritual awakening works towards enabling women to achieve their highest spiritual potential, 'the contemplative side of feminism concentrates on states of consciousness and deep mystical process at work in women's struggle for equality. A woman's inner life and freedom to pursue the mystical centre of her being are integral to her self-worth, dignity, and empowerment'.[18] Women's experience of illness creates the conditions for a unique contemplative feminism which is, as yet, unexplored in feminist spirituality.

A contributing factor to women's spiritual oppression has been the indoctrination of a notion of God as male, external and judgemental, a model somewhat emulated by the medical profession. Maria Harris has argued that for women to spiritually awaken, it is necessary for them to jettison this false idea of God. The study of the women's narratives has uncovered similarities between their journeys through invisible illnesses and the mystical journey of Teresa of Avila to the centre of the castle: 'As the soul advances towards the center of its castle, consciousness moves from oppression to freedom, from human love to divine love, and from doubt

---

16   Ibid., 18.
17   Ibid., 22.
18   Ibid., 62.

to certainty'.[19] Such a journey means that embedded medical attitudes violate not only the biological health, but also the spiritual core of those struggling with invisible illnesses.

Gordon Lynch, Professor of Theology at the University of Kent, has analysed the changing patterns of modern religion in Britain. In *The New Spirituality* (2007), Lynch theorised that there is an emergence of a different kind of spirituality in which seekers attempt to jettison this patriarchal form of religion and search for a religious practice that they believe to be more authentic, liberating and more appropriate to contemporary theories.[20]

## Narrative as Facilitator of Spiritual Awakening

Diverse disciplines explored in this study have highlighted the significance of narrative for human flourishing. The capacity of narrative to restore the dignity of the patient in medicine emerged as a theme throughout the study. Arthur Kleinman and Rita Charon have argued in favour of the inclusion of narrative methods as a central component in medical practice. In a similar vein, Maria Harris has argued that narrative as an educational intervention facilitates women to spiritually awaken, to explore their inner world, befriending what has been shown, and integrating it into the psyche.

In the psychotherapeutic method *psychosynthesis*, Roberto Assagioli developed a narrative approach to enable the spiritual unfoldment of the human person. He recognised that the introspection facilitated by the attentive listening to a person's narrative, afforded in psychotherapy, could enable the person to disidentify from body sensations, feelings and thoughts, such as those that arise in illness situations, and thus facilitate awakening in the depths of the human spirit beyond the illness. Finally, in the history of mysticism, Teresa of Avila's lifetime search for a confessor

19   Ibid., 108.
20   G. Lynch, *The New Spirituality: An Introduction to Progressive Belief in the Twenty-First Century* (London; New York: I. B. Tauris, 2007), 10.

who would understand the distinctive depth of her spiritual journey as a woman testifies to the importance of telling one's story as a path to spiritual unfoldment. With the frequent absence of such a confessor, Teresa used spiritual autobiography as a tool to narrate and to process her innermost thoughts and experiences.

Participants in this study had shared their narratives with friends with similar illnesses who had encountered similar disbelief and who were able to offer unconditional positive regard. This support was deemed a crucial step for the participants on their spiritual awakening journey. In some cases narratives of illness were facilitated by support groups, formal and informal, and in other examples, on the telephone.

As discussed previously, Beverly Lanzetta has argued that the listening ear is a healing resource in itself which enables a process whereby the woman recognises the effects of the violation of her body and spirit as female and is an invaluable contribution to spiritual awakening.

The listening ear provides healing not only for the narrator but for the listener as well, Julia Kristeva has argued. In facing up to the vulnerability of those who are marginalised, a deeper understanding and meaning-making of the human being can take place in the listener. Acknowledging vulnerability in the human being brings about the capacity for 'a perpetual re-birth of the subject, if and only if this vulnerability is recognized'.[21]

Both Julia Kristeva and Susan Wendell have addressed the yawning gulf between those who are well and those who are sick. Kristeva perceived an *abyss* of separation between the world of the disabled from the world of the able-bodied. Kristeva wrote, 'And it is urgent to create *messengers* between these "two merciless worlds": one of disability with its sufferings and its protective but also aggravating isolation; the other, a society of performance, success, competition, pleasure, and spectacle that "doesn't want to know"'.[22] Narrative and attentive listening to the narrative of the ill person enables the construction of a bridge over this yawning chasm.

21    Kristeva, *Hatred and Forgiveness*, 41.
22    Ibid., 39.

## Spirit Speaks Through Illness: A Call for a New Medical Paradigm

A recurring theme throughout the study is a call for a paradigm in medicine which can practically and effectively enable the person who is suffering to feel respected and validated. The void has somewhat been addressed by narrative medicine and by the discourses of the medical humanities. The praiseworthy efforts and achievements of the medical humanities endeavour, however, could be augmented by ideas from Roberto Assagioli's psychosynthesis model as well as the theories of process oriented psychotherapy developed by Arnold Mindell. These theories point to an opportunity for a new paradigm of medicine which would not merely enable the individual to feel validated, but to discern a new voice, the voice of the illness, that might indeed be beckoning the individual who is suffering towards a new way of being. In addition, the voice of illness bears wisdom for society in relation to the environment, social justice and new possibilities for health care.

Although Mindell is not a philosopher nor does he claim to be a phenomenologist in the tradition of Husserl, his work is inadvertently true to Husserl's aim to reach the essence of experience, identifying with that essence and giving it expression.

Feeling into and identifying with one miniscule sensation can take up a vast amount of time in an hour-long process session. In another session I worked with a sensation that I described as the mist, it relates to an extreme and frightening experience of the mind going blank or foggy, and is associated with ME. This session facilitated not just an expansion of consciousness but more energy to operate in the world. Mindell claimed that by generating keen awareness of symptoms we access 'a central experience found in many spiritual traditions, an experience of oneness where things get done without you "doing" them.'[23]

Mindell envisions a medicine of the future, *rainbow medicine*, embracing the allopathic approach and integrating, 'physics, psychology, and

---

23   A. Mindell, *The Quantum Mind and Healing: How to Listen and Respond to Your Body's Symptoms* (Charlottesville, VA: Hampton Roads Pub. Co., 2004), 24.

biology with the wisdom of humankind's earliest religions.'[24] In rainbow medicine, when symptoms strike, 'you are neither ill nor well, young nor old, but simply on a path, of whose intent you are not yet conscious.'[25]

Mindell compares a symptom to a *koan*. In Zen traditions a *koan* is a paradoxical or seemingly senseless statement such as, 'listen to the sound of one hand clapping'. In this sense, symptoms are seen as constructive in nature not to be dismissed without being listened to at a deeper level. Illness, Mindell posited 'may be the moment you have been secretly waiting for; the challenge to contact your deepest nature. In a way your symptoms may lead to some form of enlightenment.'[26]

Psycho-spiritual researcher Rosemarie Anderson viewed human wounds as sites of hospitality to transcendent wisdom and has argued that these wounds can be transformed to sources of inspiration for others. A context for healing which would enable people who are ill to be treated not merely in a respectful manner, but as bearers of radical wisdom for humanity which is being birthed through the illness, constitutes the overarching call of this study. The testimonies of the participants in this study who have faced illness, disbelief and marginalisation, yet who have been able to contextualise their experiences as opportunities for spiritual awakening, have corroborated the theories of Beverly Lanzetta and Maria Harris that women can spiritually awaken by navigating the dark night of the soul as Teresa of Avila had done nearly five centuries ago.


## Illness as a Portal to Creativity and Wisdom


Henri Ellenberger was a psychiatrist and a criminologist who became Professor of Criminology at the Université de Montréal. He was also the first historiographer of psychiatry. In his book *The Discovery of the*

---

24    Ibid., 20.
25    Ibid.
26    Ibid.

*Unconsc*ious (1970), he explored the notion of the *creative illness* as experienced by Freud and Jung. Between 1894 and 1900, Sigmund Freud (1856–1939) suffered an illness which he himself labelled *neurasthenia*. Ellenberger proposes that this was a *creative illness.*[27]

> It occurs in various settings and is to be found among shamans, among the mystics of various religions, in certain philosophers and creative writers … A creative illness follows a period of intense pre-occupation with an idea and search for a certain truth. It is a polymorphous condition that can take the shape of depression, neurosis, psychosomatic ailments, or even psychosis. Whatever the symptoms they are felt as painful, if not agonising, by the subject with alternating periods of alleviation and worsening. Throughout the illness the subject never loses the thread of his dominating preoccupation.[28]

Ellenberger's description echoes the language of the *dark night*. A further characteristic of creative illness which he explored was the feeling of isolation experienced by the subject. He noted that the termination of the illness is usually rapid and accompanied by a phase of exhilaration. 'The subject emerges from his ordeal with a permanent transformation in his personality and the conviction that he has discovered a great truth or a new spiritual world.'[29]

Concepts such as 'creative illness' bring together in a challenging framework ideas which previously may have existed in opposition. Illness may provide the conditions which make invention possible.

Chronic ill health may set the stage for the inventive process, the stages of which have been delineated by inventor Joseph Rossman (1899–1972). He demarcated seven stages of the inventive process which may also illumine the process of creativity emerging in illness. Rossman, a psychologist and chemical engineer, who worked as a patent examiner at the US patent office, in 1931 conducted a pioneering study of 710 inventors in order to identify their personality traits. He published his findings in *The*

---

27  H. Ellenberger, *The Discovery of the Unconscious: The History and Evolution of Dynamic Psychiatry* (New York: Basic Books, 1970), 447.
28  Ibid.
29  Ibid., 448.

*Psychology of the Inventor*.[30] The seven steps for the creative model which he proposed were: observation of a difficulty; analysis of that difficulty; survey of all available information; formulation of all objective solutions; critical analysis of these solutions for their advantages and disadvantages; birth of the new idea – the invention, and lastly, experimentation to test out the most promising solution, and the selection and perfection of the final embodiment by some or all of the previous steps.[31]

Medical sociologist Arthur Frank writes and lectures on illness narratives. He argues that the ultimate creativity arising out of illness is the letting go of a way of being in the world and taking the opportunity to create a new life. In his book *At the Will of the Body* (2002), he affirmed: 'illness takes away parts of your life but in doing so it gives you the opportunity to choose the life you will lead, as opposed to living out the one you have simply accumulated over the years.'[32]

Lecturer in the psychology of art at Saybrook University in San Francisco, Tobi Zausner, penned *When Walls Become Doorways: Creativity and the Transforming Illness*.[33] Zausner's publication focused on the transformative power of illness, using the examples of the lives of great artists whose physical disorders led to life transformation. One of the cases she used to illustrate her point was Nancy Fried, an American artist who had suffered cancer four times from 1986 to 1990. Fried expressed her trauma through her art as a way of coping. She created sculptures of herself with one breast. Her work became so famous that some of her sculptures were purchased by the Metropolitan Museum of Art in New York.

Zausner contended that the wall of illness became a doorway of possibility for many artists and this assertion embraced her own personal experience. She traced how the notion of the transforming illness is found

---

30   J. Rossman, *The Psychology of the Inventor: A Study of the Patentee*, new and rev. (Washington, DC: Inventors Publishing, 1931).

31   Ibid., 57.

32   A. Frank, *At the Will of the Body: Reflections on Illness*, 1st Mariner Books edn (Boston, MA: Houghton Mifflin, 2002), 1.

33   T. Zausner, *When Walls Become Doorways: Creativity and the Transforming Illness*, 1st edn (New York: Harmony Books, 2006).

throughout human history. Zausner cited Mircea Eliade, a scholar of comparative religions, who had found that 'shamans are only able to access their full abilities after recovering from an illness that transforms them.'[34]

Zausner defined what she meant by a transforming illness as 'a time of poor health that profoundly alters your work, your outlook, and your life ... It can take many forms, but whether the transforming illness is a single episode of poor health or a chronic condition, things are never the same afterward.'[35] She argued that illness can be viewed as a period of chaos, referring to chaos theory and the work of Illya Prigogine, who won the 1977 Nobel Prize in chemistry. Prigogine had described chaos as a state of turbulence in which things may appear disordered but in fact already have an inherent structure that can produce a new order.[36,37] 'The transforming illness also looks disordered, but it, too, holds the seeds for a new existence,' Zausner claimed.

Tobi Zausner proffered that creativity is not only the domain of artists but part of being human: 'Every choice we make in life is based on a decision, and the decision is a creative response to the conditions at the moment.'[38] Ill people through their responses to the circumstances of their everyday suffering have an opportunity to create their lives anew. Zausner's notion that creativity is not merely the preserve of gifted artists, but fundamental to every human being, echoes the theory of Abraham Maslow.

Philip Sandblom, who held the position of Professor of Surgery at Lund University in Sweden, asserted that suffering has a long history of being associated with artistic creativity. Sandblom was an art aficionado whose private collection included masterpieces from Renoir, Picasso, Matisse and other masters. In his book *Creativity and Disease: How Illness*

34   Ibid., 7.
35   Ibid., 8.
36   Ibid., 10.
37   I. Prigogine and I. Stengers, *Order out of Chaos: Man's New Dialogue with Nature* (Toronto: Bantam Books, 1984).
38   Zausner, *When Walls Become Doorways*, 18.

*affects literature, art and music*,[39] Sandblom inquired into the ways in which diseases contributed to the creativity of outstanding artists including Dostoyevsky, Chopin, Munch, Nietzsche, Beethoven, Chekhov and Sylvia Plath. Sandblom wrote, 'my studies of the lives of artists have led me to conclude that many have been influenced by disease and thus I understand that the view ... that healthy, harmonious individuals often lack the spur that incites "the demoniac ones" to heights of genius'.[40]

Sandblom has argued that disease, by preventing other activity, may be a factor that awakens artistic creativity in the sufferer, and offers the opportunity to develop it.[41] He pointed out that Vivaldi had been ordained a priest but, due to asthma was unable to fulfil that calling. Instead he bequeathed great music. Dostoyevsky exploited his experience of epilepsy in fiction. Five of his characters, including Prince Myshkin in *The Idiot*, suffered epileptic attacks.[42]

Sandblom profiled Keats's distress whilst suffering from tuberculosis and how, during his final years, Keats had reflected on the relationship between disease and creativity. Sandblom quoted Keats: 'How astonishing does the chance of leaving the world impress a sense of its natural beauties on us ... I muse with the greatest affection on every flower I have known from my infancy – their shapes and colours are as new to me as if I had just created them with a superhuman fancy'.[43]

In addition, Sandblom noted that Matisse had started painting after appendicitis interrupted a legal career. Sandblom was also impressed that Beethoven composed *Pastoral Symphony* while suffering from a deafness which agonised him. He cited Beethoven, 'I felt unable to leave this world before I had created what had been assigned to me; and so I endured this miserable life – really miserable'.[44] While it is not a universal outcome

---

39    P. Sandblom, *Creativity and Disease: How Illness Affects Literature, Art, and Music*, rev. 7th/1st paperback (New York: Marion Boyars, 1992).
40    Ibid., 26.
41    Ibid., 28.
42    Ibid., 84.
43    Ibid., 152.
44    Ibid., 123.

that illness generates artistic creativity, the outstanding examples of such an outcome are inspirational for this research.

## Illness, Solitude and Spiritual Awakening

This study has established the manner in which one of the prime challenges of illness is solitude. Metaphysical poet, John Donne (1572–1632), who was challenged by numerous periods of illness, declared solitude to be the greatest misery of illness.[45] Isolation ensuing from loss of friendship is exacerbated for women with invisible illnesses because of the associated mental health interpretations, marking out invisible illness as distinctive from other chronic illnesses. Solitude, on the other hand, was a major contributing factor to a high level of self-awareness evident in the narratives of the participants in the study.

Robert Grant considers the journey through trauma as the hero's journey, comparing it to Dante's *inferno*. The journey, he insisted, requires going much deeper than our collective consciousness wants us to go. Grant further claimed that there are few other ways to the Spirit other than the way of the wound: 'Due to innumerable distractions and material advantages the spiritual skin of many privileged Westerners is rarely, if ever, penetrated by life's deeper mysteries. At best, anxiety is experienced and relief immediately sought. Pain is avoided at all costs'.[46]

Whereas at one time the shaman and the healer, and their confrontations with truth, were supported in their cultures, the healing journey is now frequently undertaken alone. Grant proposed that those 'taking up the path of healing become modern-day mystics who inspire the rest of humanity to keep reaching for wholeness and the Spirit'.[47] Grant put forward an argument for a *spirituality of trauma* which would have the potential to

---

45  Donne, *The Works of John Donne*, 513.
46  Grant, *The Way of the Wound*, 9.
47  Ibid., 6.

recover what has been personally and culturally disowned. This would be a path downwards, into the dark waters of trauma as opposed to upwards towards the light. He equated trauma to shamanic initiation, 'Initiation often involves being wounded and then a long process of working through the consequences of these wounds'.[48] He based his spirituality of trauma on the journey of spiritual awakening as delineated by Evelyn Underhill, adding another phase in the beginning: shock. Shock, he theorised, comes before purgation, illumination and union. He asserted that this spirituality of trauma does not promise a cure. It is about a re-organisation of consciousness.

Grant asserted that the nature of human existence entails a constant state of being and becoming. However, the important position given to the ego in Western culture has an effect of maintaining a fixed sense of 'who I am'. Grant argued that the effect of this is to 'damn the incessant flow of being and becoming and design a once-and-for- all version of self'.[49]

Grant insisted that a key aspect of spiritual awakening through the Way of the Wound is the re-examination of one's image of God. Childhood images of God must die: 'God is often an exponential version of a judgemental or a punishing parent, or a Being who can grant any wish, attend to any need and respond to one's magical prayers .... Traumatic events are usually required before most are willing to re-examine and later revise their "images" of God'.[50]

Grant averred that the 'Profound realisations and unsettling questions, carried by every victim of trauma, are typically disowned and, by necessity, overlooked by mainstream consciousness'.[51]

Marginalisation of ill people can exacerbate their feelings of isolation. However, Grant considers the trauma of marginalisation as an opportunity for spiritual awakening:

---

48    Ibid., 8.
49    Grant, *The Way of the Wound*, 17.
50    Ibid., 9.
51    Ibid., 90.

The path of the marginalised is the path of all trauma victims. It is also the path of liberation and spiritual growth. To be marginal is to be cast out of the 'taken for granted' which in many cases is blind, sedated and thus the illusory version of reality. Social reality promises happiness in exchange for the denial and suppression of certain personal and existential truths. Acceptance of this pact severely reduces any chance of authentic development.[52]

Trauma, according to Grant, exposes the existential restlessness and completeness at the core of one's being, which the ego strives to hide: 'Victims are forced to acknowledge their limitations and impoverishments, along with a growing awareness that they cannot live without others or Spirit.'[53]

Once the ego is displaced, Grant argues, Spirit finds an opportunity to enter. The person is forced to understand that life involves a series of losses, and that riches are inherent in every loss. Citing the philosopher Heidegger, Grant argued that the 'taken for granted' is not usually examined, until it breaks down. On a website 'blog' titled *Trauma, Addiction and Spirituality*, Grant pronounced that trauma provides an opportunity to walk a path 'that spiritual adepts have been walking for thousands of years – albeit alone, without maps or guides and shaken to the core.'[54]

The importance of solitude as a fundamental constituent on the path of spiritual awakening, and as a prerequisite for empowerment, has been noted by Bernadette Flanagan.[55] Flanagan has investigated the importance of solitude for the spiritual lives of five women spiritual innovators across history: Syncletica, Moninne, Mary of Oignies, Angela Merici and Nano Nagle, and a cohort of modern-day women spiritual seekers. She conceptualises solitude as 'the place where it is possible to discover the very essence of one's own being, what is utterly original and uniquely woven

---

52    Ibid., 34.
53    Ibid., 19.
54    <http://in-sigththerapy.blogspot.ie/2013/06/trauma-addiction-and-spirituality.html>. Accessed 15 October 2015.
55    B. Flanagan, *Embracing Solitude: Women and New Monasticism* (Eugene, OR: Resource Publications, 2013).

into the fabric of one's being'.[56] This construct echoes the deeper solitude experience of participants of this study.

Flanagan has noted a high level of self-awareness in visionary leaders. The findings of this research testify to an impressive level of self-awareness in the cohort of women interviewed. 'In general,' she has proffered, 'visionary leaders have more self-awareness and a greater capacity for reflective attunement than many others, and they tend to lead from the inside out .... Indeed in leadership science today the capacity for solitude is perceived as a leadership metacompetence'.[57] The women interviewed in this study who faced invisible illnesses have developed a leadership metacompetence as well as a metacompetence for resilience.

56    Ibid., 4.
57    Ibid., xxv.

# Seven-stage Model of Spiritual Awakening amongst Women with Chronic Invisible Illnesses

While it is not possible to break down the spiritual journey of a human being into precise chronological stages, this seven-stage spiral model constitutes an endeavour to create a prototype of the spiritual awakening journey of women who experience spiritual awakening in chronic invisible illness. Evelyn Underhill expressed reservations about any classification or mapping of the landscape of the soul, stating that: 'The creative impulse in the world, so far as we are aware of it, appears upon ultimate analysis to be free and original, not bound and mechanical'.[1] She insisted that her characterisations would be construed as, 'only answering loosely and generally to experiences which seldom present themselves in so rigid and unmixed a form'.[2] In a similar fashion, this model is offered as a heuristic device. Some of the characteristics of one stage may appear in another stage. Stages are analogous to waypoints on a journey, each one representing an aspect or a phase of the woman's mystical path through chronic invisible illness. The model is grounded in a deeper consideration of the themes which emerged from the analysis of all of the narratives, in conjunction with the literature reviewed earlier. The model indicates the main authors associated with each stage and hence acts as a useful framework for deeper study (see Figure 2).

---

1    Underhill, *Mysticism*, 167.
2    Ibid., 168.

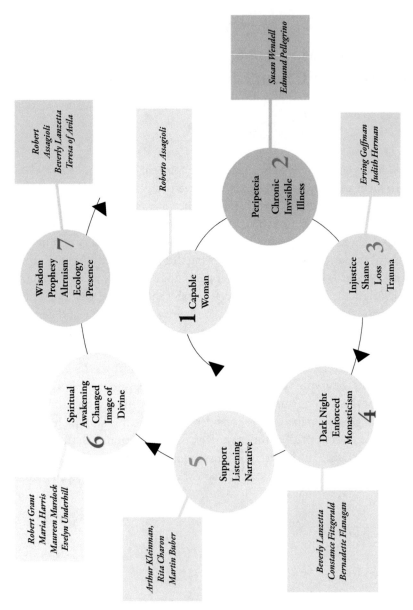

Figure 2.  Seven-stage model of spiritual awakening amongst women with invisible/
contested illnesses

## Seven-stage Model Explained

The seven stages are named according to the qualities or characteristics associated with that stage:

1.   Capable Woman
2.   Chronic Invisible Illness
3.   Injustice, Shame, Loss and Trauma
4.   Dark Night and Enforced Monasticism
5.   Listening, Support and Narrative Medicine
6.   Spiritual Awakening – Changed Image of the Divine
7.   Wisdom, Prophesy, Altruism, Ecology, and Presence

*Stage 1: Capable Woman*

The first stage in the spiral has been titled 'Capable Woman'. At this initial stage of the journey, the woman feels relatively in control of her life. She has a good career, perhaps in a steady relationship and is optimistic about the future. Key theorists associated with this initial stage include Roberto Assagioli, one of the originators of transpersonal theory. He argued that for the individual whose life runs smoothly, there is little attention to matters of Spirit. 'He takes life as it comes and does not worry about the problems of its meaning; he devotes himself to the satisfaction of his personal desires; he seeks enjoyment of the senses and endeavours to become rich and satisfy his ambitions.'[3] If one applies Assagioli's subpersonality theory, it would suggest that at this stage Capable Woman's 'I' is identified with an unexamined 'hard worker' subpersonality, as her sense of identity is bound up with her career.

   For Sally, the Capable Woman stage was a bearer of 'great excitement and possibilities galore, ... I was in every paper I was on the telly a couple of times it is just a surreal, very surreal time actually suddenly your creations

3    Assagioli, *Psychosynthesis: A Manual of Principles and Techniques*, 40.

that you're making ... are out there in magazines.' In my own case, I was forging ahead with a career in television journalism in London, as my 'I' was unconsciously identified with a need to prove that I was intelligent.


*Stage 2: Chronic Invisible Illness*

In the second stage the 'peripeteia' occurs – the event which changes the woman's life – chronic invisible illness. She may experience numerous physical symptoms which leave her weak and ill, yet doctors are unable to establish the cause of the illness with standard laboratory tests. Her identity as a capable woman is challenged and she endures the four losses which prompted Edmund Pellegrino towards establishing medical humanities: the loss of freedom of action; the loss of freedom to make rational choices; the loss of freedom from the power of others, and the loss of a sense of the integrity of the self.[4] In addition to these four losses enumerated by Pellegrino, invisible illness may also bring in its wake the wounds of loss of credibility, friendship, and, ultimately, the supports typically expected in times of illness. At this phase of chronic invisible illness, intimate relationships may also break up. Susan Wendell, feminist and professor emerita of philosophy, whose career suffered because of ME, has critiqued feminism for having little consolation for women in this position: 'Good feminists, like good women everywhere, are supposed to give 'til it hurts; everyone is supposed to feel exhausted and overworked, so why should I be the exception? "We" don't have time to be ill, to coddle ourselves.'[5]

Julia, the former nurse who participated in this study, spoke poignantly about the amplified nature of the effects on her life of the disbelief of medical personnel. She could not comprehend that a profession, to which she had dedicated her life, would disbelieve her when she developed electro-hypersensitivity: 'I was ... dead really to what I knew ....' For Angela, her peripeteia was brought on by TB which remained 'invisible' to the

---

4    Spicker and Ratzan, 'Ars Medicina Et Conditio Humana Edmund D. Pellegrino, M. D., on His 70th Birthday', 327.
5    Wendell, *The Rejected Body*, 1996, 4.

medical gaze for many years: 'It was totally traumatic to be transitioning into womanhood and transitioning into menstruation, and at the same time manifesting like a horrible illness ... it took all of my 20s, and half of my 30s, before I finally got someone to figure out what was wrong with me.'

## Stage 3: Injustice, Shame, Loss and Trauma

The third stage incorporates the woman's experiences of injustice, shame, loss, and trauma – an experience of alienation and stigma. Lack of validation by the medical profession often results in lack of belief of friends, family and associates. Those with invisible illnesses may also feel alienated in the media as journalists make insensitive comments about how those with contested illnesses may be imagining they are sick, or feigning it. Erving Goffman argued that stigmatisation is a process which spoils one's sense of normal identity.[6] Lack of validation by the medical profession rendered it difficult for the majority of the participants to negotiate the first stage of recovery from trauma delineated by renowned trauma theorist, Judith Herman. She argued that the establishment of safety is brought about by attending to the basic needs of the body, including 'attention to basic health needs, regulation of body functions such as sleep, eating and exercise'.[7] Herman further argued that sufferers of all forms of trauma need a supportive environment in order to be able to speak out about their pain. In the absence of any strong political movement which would validate their trauma, the process of forgetting is inevitable.[8]

Angela's sense of alienation was evident as she expressed frustration about having to explain her illness to others 'you don't know how to explain it to them because you ... don't know what the hell is happening to you ... you can't explain it to anybody, let alone yourself, and so there you are with like all your own questions and everybody else's questions ... they are all pointing the finger.'

6    Goffman, *Stigma*, 160.
7    Herman, *Trauma and Recovery*, 160.
8    Ibid., 9.

*Stage 4: Dark Night and Enforced Monasticism*

The fourth stage is a dark night of the soul, a stage of 'enforced monasticism'; much time is spent alone. While most of the old friendships have disintegrated, new friends have yet to emerge. Here, the woman with invisible illnesses is reliant on her own inner resources; however, the wisdom which would enable her to make meaning of her experience, in a healthy way, has not yet emerged. Many hours are spent perhaps gazing through the window – reading or watching TV demands energy and concentration that is not available to her. Constance Fitzgerald has argued that every human being experiences impasse or dark night, a condition of stagnation which defies fixing with the logical rational mind. Fitzgerald has argued that spirituality itself is in a state of impasse, as old patriarchal images of God no longer work, but no satisfactory image or structure has come into being. In a similar vein, orthodox medicine has little to offer the woman with invisible illness. Fitzgerald affirmed the wisdom of yielding to impasse, 'responding with full consciousness of one's suffering in the impasse yet daring to believe that new possibilities, beyond immediate vision, can be given.'[9] This stage is reflected in Beverly Lanzetta's 'via feminina', grounded in the crystalline castle framework of Teresa of Avila, and which proposed a feminist mystical theology of healing for women.[10] This is a type of via negativa, apophasis or undoing, a negation, or a criticism of patriarchy in the lives and interactions of women and men. It encompasses a period of letting go of untruths about women, followed by a period of reintegration of spiritual wisdom and soul healing. She argues that women benefit from such a healing process which moves them from oppression and illness to liberation and healing. Teresa of Avila dealt with the dismissive behaviour meted out to her in a male-dominated Church and felt the pain of female embodiment, but her gift in return was an inflow of divine wisdom. She gained the strength to understand this cruelty as a 'desecration of the holy'.[11]

9     Fitzgerald, 'Impasse and Dark Night', 289–90.
10    Lanzetta, *Radical Wisdom*, 16.
11    Ibid., 125.

A dark night of misunderstanding is a feature of the chronic invisible illness experience, as often the illness is diagnosed as depression. This diagnosis led to women in this study feeling misjudged, and had implications for the type of medications prescribed. Sally stated: 'The doctors several times have offered me anti-depressants but I don't actually feel depressed, I feel sad but I don't actually feel depressed.' Mary Rose, with the benefit of hindsight, discerned that the enforced solitude and the dark night of misunderstanding associated with her illness as having been a catalyst for spiritual growth. 'Our way of life has become meditative', she stated, 'because we can't put up with the hurly burly, it makes us more receptive to Spirit ... you end up re-creating yourself, you become a new creation.'

*Stage 5: Listening, Support, and Narrative Medicine*

This fifth stage represents the development of new friendships, or connections with others, which are life-giving; often these connections are generated with others who have had their own invisible illness experiences. Here, the woman with invisible illness is able to tell her story to individuals who believe her. She feels listened to on a deep level, and feels affirmed; a new trust in life is birthed. Key to this phase is the healing power of narrative, as an 'I and Thou' quality characterises the relationship.[12]

As a medical anthropologist, Arthur Kleinman has studied the way in which illness is socially constructed, arguing that 'there are normal ways of being ill (ways that our society regards as appropriate) as well as anomalous ways'.[13] When an illness is contested, telling one's narrative is especially therapeutic. Kleinman has argued that telling one's story of illness has an empowering effect, asserting that patients may benefit by doctors being able to listen to their patients like amateur ethnographers, to the detail of the terrain of the patient's bodily symptoms. He has lamented that

---

12    Martin Buber, *I and Thou* (New York: Scribner, 1970).
13    Kleinman, *The Illness Narratives*, 5.

medical training 'inculcates values and behaviours that are antithetical to the humane care of patients.'[14]

Rita Charon of New York University's School of Medicine, who initiated formal education in 'narrative medicine', coaches medical professionals in deep listening skills for the purpose of attending to narratives of illness. She asserted that the 'self' of the doctor is her most powerful therapeutic instrument, and that doctors must work toward their own self-awareness in order to be able to listen attentively to the patient. Charon argued that narratology was often the 'silent partner to human beings as they make and mark meaning, coping with the contingencies of moral and mental life.'[15] She stressed that medicine has lagged behind other disciplines where a shift towards narrative has taken place, 'challenging scholars and practitioners from religious studies to psychoanalysis to police work to concentrate not just on the facts, but on the situations in which the facts are told.'[16]

Sharon, a participant in this study, wept as she recalled the healing value of one her new friendships, with a woman she met through a support group's online 'chatroom' who rang her every morning at about 11.00 'without fail' from Germany: 'and it's that that got me out of bed and I have got such gratitude for this woman, and she is suffering way more than me still, and yet she had the compassion to do that for me ... these people we are all walking in the same shoes, we are all the same ....'

### Stage 6: Spiritual Awakening – Changed Image of the Divine

The sixth stage, representing an awakening to a new level of consciousness, corresponds with the first stage of Evelyn Underhill's five stages in the mystical journey, and also with the first step of Maria Harris's seven-step 'dance of the Spirit'. Underhill described this stage as a disturbance in the equilibrium of the self, causing a shift in the field of consciousness to a higher level, a 'removal of the centre of interest from the subject to an

---

14    Ibid., 257.
15    Charon, *Narrative Medicine*, 40.
16    Ibid., 11.

object now brought into view: the necessary beginning of any process of transcendence.'[17] Harris theorised on the significance of this alteration for the inner life: 'Layers, crusts, and shells which may have been built up over years become brittle, break apart, and begin to disappear .... And a realization dawns that a personal daystar has begun to shine, giving us light.'[18]

Like Harris, Jungian psychologist, Maureen Murdock, has argued that women, in order to awaken, must travel through the journey of their personal suffering. She correlated this journey through suffering with the mythical 'descent to the underworld', theorising that it is concerned with reclaiming the rejected feminine aspect, reclaiming the Goddess; Murdock claims that the women who undertake reclamation of the rejected feminine are rediscovering the lost soul of their culture.[19]

Trauma theorist, Robert Grant, has asserted that a key aspect of spiritual awakening through what he termed 'the way of the wound' is the re-examination of one's image of God, arguing that childhood images of God must die. 'God is often an exponential version of a judgemental or a punishing parent, or a Being who can grant any wish, attend to any need and respond to one's magical prayers .... Traumatic events are usually required before most are willing to re-examine and later revise their "images" of God'.[20]

Rachel, who had been identified with her 'scholarship girl' sub-personality, and had gained a sense of identity from her teaching profession, described how, during her long dark night of suffering, a paranormal vision of a beautiful light awakened her to a new understanding of the unconditional nature of pure divine love, bringing her new freedom from her attachment to her career identity. This mystical experience awakened her to a new insight, and a new image of the divine, which had a profound effect on her life, 'that's what the light told me ... that love is there for you it doesn't have to be merited.'

17    Underhill, *Mysticism: The Nature and Development of Spiritual Consciousness*, 176.
18    Harris, *Dance of the Spirit*, 5.
19    Murdock, *The Heroine's Journey*, 9.
20    Grant, *The Way of the Wound*, 9.

*Stage 7: Wisdom, Prophesy, Altruism, Ecology, and Presence*

This seventh stage represents the integration of the rewards the woman has reaped as a result of her chronic invisible illness experience. She has now assimilated into her personality fruits of the higher unconscious, as depicted in the oval diagram of Assagioli. These boons include: self-awareness, wisdom, kindness, compassion, a new more authentic form of self-confidence, intuitive abilities, and serenity. She has a stronger sense of social justice and ecology and the unity rather than the division of mind and body. From her isolation experience, she has gone some way towards healing the repression of the feminine, which, Lanzetta has argued, mirrors the most fundamental tensions such as, 'ancient division in intellectual history between body and soul, matter and spirit, human and divine, humanity and the natural world'.[21] This division, Lanzetta has stressed, is responsible for violence against women and other subjugated groups and 'is at the core of our cultural pathology'.[22] Reflecting the journey of Teresa of Avila, the woman at this stage of the spiral has completed a spiral round of the psycho-spiritual journey, the inward journey towards the Self, the divine essence which is a movement into self-knowledge.[23] Teresa exemplified a strong sense of self-worth through an inner journey and a dark night in which she suffered misogyny from confessors who dismissed her experience of the spiritual life. Despite the Inquisition, she wrote and taught her contemplative path, based on her inner experience. Teresa's journey convinced Lanzetta that the mystic's path has a lot to offer women who suffer from oppression today, 'this mystical emptiness of self initiates an unreserved responsibility in which our mystics reclaim their dignity as women and articulate a new feminine way of liberation for themselves and for others'.[24]

Typically of the research participants, Angela claimed that her illness has made her more altruistic and, furthermore, that the experience of

---

21    Lanzetta, *Radical Wisdom*, 10–11.
22    Ibid.
23    Welch, *Spiritual Pilgrims*, 3.
24    Lanzetta, *Radical Wisdom*, 118.

being very ill is something she must carry with her for the good of society, 'it's like as if I need to be anchored in the experience that my illness has given me, because it opens me, it makes me a kinder person, it makes me a more aware person, it allows me to be more attuned to others' needs, it has trained me in the needs for acceptance, and if you don't accept in life you are going nowhere, it's like acceptance is just a cornerstone of existence ... if you can gather all of your existence and all of your life and all of your experience into your heart and say yes to it, I think you are doing yourself a great service and you are also doing the planet a great service.'

After this final stage, another round of the spiral begins, because the chronic invisible illness situation continues indefinitely. The seven-stage process will witness, however, greater awareness as the woman with invisible illness re-enters the Capable Woman stage; in addition, she has integrated the boons of the heroine's journey.

# CHAPTER 8

# Empowering the Marginalised

The precise scale of the problem of chronic invisible/contested illness is unknown. The burgeoning collection of international websites concerning chronic fatigue syndrome, fibromyalgia, Lyme disease, multiple chemical sensitivity, invisible illnesses and contested illnesses would suggest that the issue is here to stay. An awareness week for people with invisible illnesses is publicised, for example, on the San Diego based website titled *Invisible Illness Awareness Week*.[1] In its disciplinary foundations, this is the first study to draw on psycho-spiritual theory to identify the steps on the journey of spiritual awakening in women with chronic invisible/contested illnesses. The research approach used resulted in an understanding of the predicament of women with chronic invisible illnesses that hinder their ability to live normal lives, but who are not believed. The findings have significant implications for the understanding of how the phenomenon affects their lives in their inner world of meaning-making and in the practicalities of how it affects how they benefit or not from the care of other people. The seven-stage spiral model, the first conceptual map of inner growth occurring as a consequence of invisible/contested illness experience, provides a unique window on the phenomenon of how marginalised people can spiritually awaken and become empowered. This model integrates previous research work by prominent authors in this field and offers a hopeful model of chronic invisible illness with the message that oppression and marginalisation bring with them the potential for the development of a deeper level of consciousness. Something unique has been created in this research enterprise, a fact endorsed by the absence of any prior models with which the author could compare her suggested model.

[1]    <http://invisibleillnessweek.com>. Accessed 7 August 2015.

Through weaving together existing theory on trauma and applying it to the case of chronic invisible illness, this book crafts a theory of trauma in chronic invisible illness. The extent to which trauma appeared in the narratives of the women interviewed was unexpected. Although some aspects of trauma were caused by the illness itself, the overarching source of trauma was lack of belief by the medical profession. The harrowing nature of the trauma surrounding disbelief and the organic, seamless way in which that theme developed as a thread through the categorised themes was unexpected. The manner in which not being believed by doctors – and the often insensitive way in which disbelief was communicated – had progressive detrimental consequences for the narrators, was particularly striking. This research has generated rich descriptions of a sequence of traumatic experiences sequential and consequential to not being believed. None of this material was directly and explicitly sought out by the researcher. At no time were participants asked a question such as, 'Tell me about not being believed?' This affords gravitas to the findings on disbelief. This also points to the power of this procedure for narrative research where there is minimal use of prepared questionnaires.

A further unexpected finding, still on the subject of trauma, constituted the way in which I personally experienced re-traumatisation as I worked on particular phases of the research. This trauma presented itself when 'triggered', or re-stimulated, by the material when writing my personal narrative, whilst transcribing and analysing interviews, and on reading some of the literature. The reflexive component in the methodology of the research enabled me to be mindful of the process that was occurring in my psyche, and to work with it through journaling and therapy. Romanyshyn's 'wounded researcher' archetype offered profound insight into the re-traumatising process. His theory explains why I sometimes felt grief-stricken by the marginalisation of some of the women and why at other times I felt myself, disconcertingly, in the shoes of the perpetrator of the marginalisation process, wanting to distance myself from their suffering and stigmatisation.

The quality of atmosphere I experienced during the interviews left a lasting impression. A flavour of this energy is captured to some degree in excerpts from the narratives allied to spiritual awakening; these are imbued with lightness and have a poetic quality. The reader is transported to another reality, to a transpersonal domain. In a quest for vocabulary to describe such states of consciousness, Stanislav Grof, one of the founders of the transpersonal movement, opted for the term *numinous* which he claimed was first employed by Lutheran theologian Rudolph Otto (1869–1937). *Numinous* derives from nūmen, a Latin word to denote the presence of a deity. 'The sense of numinosity', Grof elucidated, 'is based on direct apprehension of the fact that we are encountering a domain that belongs to a superior order of reality, one which is sacred and radically different from the material world.'[2] Numinosity is manifested in a manner which doesn't easily lend itself to language. It concerns a mysterious quality in the tone of the voice, a certain radiance emanating from the person, and how one feels in its presence. A supplementary unexpected finding on the topic of numinosity was the extent to which this particular numinous quality of presence was not restricted to moments when the participants were talking about the spiritual or transformative aspects of the illness, but it also permeated the whole of the narratives even as they spoke of suffering, negation and rejection.

A further unexpected finding is constituted in the way in which I have personally experienced spiritual awakening as a result of this academic undertaking. The years invested in the project have witnessed a period of my own growing alignment with gifts from the higher unconscious, including patience, love, compassion and desire for social justice for women who have had the experiences discussed in the book. The research project has facilitated the creation of a wider concept of illness which integrates a view of illness as socially constructed from the religio-cultural paradigms which are inherited and transmitted unconsciously. The study has afforded me a new confidence born out of a sense of hermeneutical justice which has been provided by the educational journey of the study. A longstanding belief in the value of illness as a force for good in the world has been affirmed and supported by the work of scholars whose theories have been incorporated in this study.

2    S. Grof, *Psychology of the Future: Lessons from Modern Consciousness Research* (New York: SUNY Press, 2000), 210.

This research set out to explore the nature of the phenomenon of spiritual awakening in specific types of chronic illness experience with a specific population in a specific socio-cultural setting. African men living with AIDS in Malawi would have a different experience. It deliberately recruited individuals with an interest in personal development and in spirituality – these interests engender an awareness of the internal world and perhaps willingness to dialogue with some fluency about spirituality. Thus a bias existed in the sample from the beginning due to participants' interest in spirituality. It was therefore almost inevitable that no participants voiced becoming irrevocably embittered by the illness nor did any of them state that no growth had resulted from their illness experiences.

This research adopted Martin Buber's '*I* and *Thou*' ethic in its encounters with research participants. This implied treating participants with ultimate respect. The research encounter was held at a location, time and surrounding suited to interviewees and also a location which would be favourable for participants telling their story in a relaxed manner. With one exception, the location of the interview was the home of the participant. Serious debilitating illness rendered it difficult for appointments to take place. Two of the participants were available for brief episodes of time by telephone but not in person. Due to the unpredictable nature of their illnesses, those two people were reluctant to make an appointment for a personal visit from me. One implication for the research of such circumstances was a lack of homogenous criteria in respect of locations or circumstances for all of the interviews. It could be alleged that this could have affected the research outcome. It would be difficult, however, to propose an alternative solution that would be respectful of the '*I* and *Thou*' attitude, which implies respect for the relationship. Ultimately it is the relationship that enables the revelation of spirit in the narratives of the participants.

In a similar vein the research encounter did not involve a questionnaire or a strict protocol of questions. Each participant was asked to tell her story of illness. The research encounter was designed to resemble as closely as possible what might constitute a typical conversational encounter between this *wounded researcher* who has health issues, and the participants, woman to woman, over a cup of tea. Any deviation from the type of circumstances where spirituality and the inner life might normally be discussed was avoided. Therefore hotel lobbies, for example, were not considered as potential locations. Privacy and familiarity were prerequisites for the comfort necessary to begin to speak about the inner life, loss and spirituality. It could be argued by sceptics that the limitations caused by lack of a list of questions deemed the research open to manipulation by the researcher. Conversely any such list or artificial structure would negate the conditions necessary for this researcher for the creation of safe space for spirit to emerge.

Participants of this study narrated their experiences retrospectively. Knowledge gathered in this study could be enriched by longitudinal research, perhaps over a ten-year period. Such an exercise could involve a blend of journal keeping on the part of participants and periodic interviews. This type of research would enable a clearer and richer picture to emerge of the nature of trauma experienced in the present moment, and likewise a more nuanced depiction of the nature of spiritual awakening as it occurs. It would also provide material for enhancing the seven-stage model presented in this study.

An attempt is being made here to lay the groundwork for further research on ways in which illness experience may act as a catalyst for spiritual awakening and growth in wisdom. Future research, quantitative and qualitative, could be conducted on the method of working with symptoms utilising the *process* method devised by Arnold Mindell which has been elucidated in this study in relation to the researcher's personal experience. Such research would examine:

- If illness and symptoms could be viewed in a more optimistic light as a result of process work.
- If meaning making in illness could be facilitated by process work.
- The degree to which spiritual awakening is enabled by process work.

This book has several potential areas for practical application. Its findings could be used to help women who have chronic invisible/contested illnesses. These women could gain a sense of hermeneutic justice and self-esteem from the insights of Kleinman, Charon, Wendell, and other theorists from diverse disciplines featured in this book who view illness and disability as socially constructed. Theories on spiritual awakening featured here point to ways in which women may be empowered by considering illness as a possible gateway to spiritual awakening. Education on the possibility of a psycho-spiritual approach to the impasse in which they find themselves could enable women to view their illness as a monastic experience, a type of via negativa, apophasis or undoing, facilitating a criticism of patriarchy and misogyny in both medicine and society. In a manner evocative of the women featured here, sixteenth-century mystic Teresa of Avila dealt with dismissive behaviour meted out to her in a male-controlled Church and felt the pain of female embodiment – she equated this kind of cruelty to a 'desecration of the holy'.[3] The idea of illness as a contemplative path offers a hopeful paradigm that this impasse may well be followed by a period of reintegration of spiritual wisdom, leading individuals from oppression and illness to liberation and healing. The findings here point to the wisdom of supporting those who are sick to take advantage of illness by reimaging a bedridden experience as a potential hermitage experience, affording self-knowledge and the shedding of false personas. The polar star question here is can there be a respectful approach devised which would facilitate those who have chronic conditions to take advantage of illness, contested in this case, as an opportunity for spiritual awakening? Such an approach could encompass contemplative theory and listening skills as taught in spiritual accompaniment training and in psycho-spiritual programmes such as psychosynthesis.

The findings should prove to be particularly valuable to the medical profession as an aid to generate amongst its members an appreciation of the benefits of phenomenology and of narrative medicine as supplementary diagnostic tools. In addition, the information in this book on the traumatising effects of doctors' disbelief could help to fashion more compassionate clinical encounters. Charon's assertion that the 'self' of the doctor is their most powerful therapeutic instrument, and that doctors must work toward their own self-awareness in order to be able to listen attentively to the patient, deserves particular attention in instances of invisible illnesses.

3    Lanzetta, 125.

Carers, family and friends, spiritual directors, and therapists of women with chronic illness conditions which are contested could gain a deeper understanding of the extent of shame, stigma and trauma experienced in such illness situations. Such an understanding could help to alleviate their possible tendencies to be perpetrators of trauma.

Theories from eminent authors in medical humanities, trauma studies, transpersonal theory, philosophy, and spirituality, here applied to women with invisible illnesses, indicate that there is a need for a new medical paradigm which would not only enable the individual to feel validated, but to acknowledge a new voice, the voice of the illness, that might indeed be beckoning the individual towards a new way of being. This voice also bears wisdom for society in relation to the environment, social justice as well as new and more humane possibilities for health care. It is hoped that this book can serve as a messenger between the world of those who are ill with contested conditions, stigmatised and marginalised – canaries still trapped in mineshafts – and an outside world which may benefit from hearing their voices.

# Appendix: Designing an Exploratory Study: Key Factors

> Being ill is not just an objective constraint imposed on a biological body part, but a systematic shift in the way the body experiences, reacts and performs tasks as a whole. The change in illness is not local but global, not external but strikes at the heart of subjectivity.[1]
>
> — HAVI CAREL

This section summarises the exploratory methodological approach employed in this research and the rationale behind its choice. Much debate has taken place since the 1960s about how, respectfully and effectively, to conduct research into the inner world of meaning-making in the human person. That debate has interacted with two branches of philosophy, ontology and epistemology, which respectively relate to questions about what constitutes the nature of reality and what is the nature of truth.[2]

Qualitative research is eminently suited to research into the experience of chronic illness. Flick et al. have argued in the Sage publication *A Companion to Qualitative Research* (2004) that from such an approach, 'a fundamentally more concrete and plastic image often emerges of what it

---

1   H. Carel, *Illness: The Cry of the Flesh*, Art of Living Series (Acumen Publishing) (Stocksfield: Acumen, 2008), 29.
2   This research is founded on a post-positivist paradigm – this approach to social science research rejects the idea that a person can see the world as it really is. It asserts that all observation is biased and underpinned by theory. Thus, the background of the individual researcher can influence what is observed. Post-positivist research practices are deemed more suitable for effecting social change than positivist methods because these practices, according to Norman Denzin and Yvonna Lincoln, lend themselves to a multiple choice of methods in order to capture as much reality as possible in any chosen field of research.

is like, from the point of view of the person concerned, to live, for example, with a chronic illness, than could be achieved by a questionnaire.'[3] Qualitative research has a capacity to describe life experiences such as illness and spiritual awakening from the inside, from the perspective of the participants in the study. The exploratory strategy employed in this study used a qualitative research framework which draws on the theories of narrative inquiry, autoethnography, intuitive inquiry, reflexivity, phenomenology, psycho-spiritual/transpersonal psychology and hermeneutics.

This project involved six key strands of inquiry. Firstly, the writing and analysis of my personal narrative of illness was undertaken in order to lay bare my own story and position in relation to illness and spiritual awakening. Jungian psychologist Robert Romanyshyn, who is a professor emeritus at Pacifica Graduate Institute, has argued in *The Wounded Researcher* that there is an ethical imperative on the part of the researcher to write down the lingering 'weight of history that needs to be spoken'.[4] He has proposed that in order for depth psychology research to be truly ethical, researchers must examine their wounded state on a continuous basis: 'Precisely because a researcher is a wounded researcher, he or she is obliged to commit himself or herself to the task of accepting responsibility for the shadow she or he casts upon the work, as well as to attend to the unfinished business in the soul of the work'.[5] The personal narrative of illness addresses the aspects of soul wounds that are intertwined and inseparable from bodily illnesses.

The second task involved relevant literature from the field of medical humanities being researched and reviewed; thirdly, discourses on spiritual awakening were examined; fourthly, a further literature review was undertaken to contextualise the key themes which emerged from the personal narrative; then, nine participants were recruited through convenience and snowball sampling, and in-depth interviews were conducted, transcribed, and analysed using thematic content analysis. The list of themes which had been generated from the personal narrative was intentionally used

---

3    U. Flick, E. Von Kardorff, and I. Steinke, *A Companion to Qualitative Research* (Thousand Oaks, CA: Sage, 2004), 5.
4    Romanyshyn, *The Wounded Researcher*, 4.
5    Ibid., 342.

as a reference point in the undertaking of the analysis of narratives of the participants. For example, a category of themes entitled *illness and trauma* occurred in the personal narrative. This theme appeared also in the narratives of the participants. This type of autoethnographic technique has been described by Heewon Chang, Professor of Organisational Leadership and Education at Eastern University in Philadelphia, as: 'a research method that enables researchers to use data from their own life stories as situated in socio-cultural contexts in order to gain an understanding of society through the unique lens of the self.'[6] Self is both a subject to look into and a lens through which to gain an understanding of a societal culture. Finally, the major themes from participants' narratives were contextualised in the literature and the results written up. By undertaking this method, the major themes which had featured in the personal narrative, together with the literature reviews they generated, became a lens through which the narratives of the participants could be examined and contextualised in a tightly focused literature selection.

This research is constructed on narrative ways of knowing. Narrative has the advantage of providing knowledge that is unique and brings together 'layers of understanding about a person, their culture and how they have created change'.[7] Arthur Frank has argued that telling one's story of illness is a way of re-drawing old maps and finding new destinations: 'Stories have to *repair* the damage that illness has done to the ill person's sense of where she is in life, and where she may be going.'[8] He acknowledges how many people who are ill feel a responsibility to the world of the well to tell their story of illness: 'Storytelling is *for* another just as much as it is for oneself.'[9] Narratives, according to Jerome Bruner, are a way in which people make meaning in their lives. Women with chronic invisible illnesses often tell their stories of illness, and of the shaming effects of not being believed,

---

6    H. Chang, *Collaborative Autoethnography*, Developing Qualitative Inquiry (Walnut Creek, CA: Left Coast Press, 2012), 18.

7    K. Etherington, 'A View of Narrative Inquiry', 2003, < http://www.cprjournal.com/docu ments/narrativeInquiry.ppt>.

8    Frank, *The Wounded Storyteller*, 53.

9    Ibid., 17.

in informal support groups, sometimes on the telephone. Such narratives act as an organising principle of authentication in their lives. The value of narrative as an agent for healing and wellbeing has been acknowledged, as previously discussed, by medical professor Rita Charon, who established the first department of narrative medicine in a medical school.

The orthodox view of illness prevailing today has its origins in an objectivist world view. Illness is considered to be able to be accounted for by physical facts alone. Havi Carel, a phenomenology philosopher at the University of Bristol has challenged this view, based on her own story: 'The description is objective (and objectifying), neutral and third personal. It excludes the first-person experience and the changes to a person's life that illness causes'.[10] Carel saw the value of phenomenology for complementing medical science by providing descriptions of the lived experience of the ill person:

> Instead of viewing illness as a local description of a particular function, phenomenology turns to the lived experience of this dysfunction. It attends to the global disruption of the habits, capacities and actions of the ill person.[11]

French philosopher Maurice Merleau-Ponty (1908–1961) is of particular interest to this research as he developed phenomenology with a special emphasis on the body after the Second World War. Merleau-Ponty, a critic of Descartian philosophy, argued that the body is the primary vehicle of knowing, and, that the body and what it perceived could not be separated from one another. He taught his philosophy against the backdrop of a French society with 'a strong tradition that takes the natural sciences as the paradigms of knowledge' going back to Descartes.[12] Much of his undertaking was concerned with mending dualistic thinking, bridging the gap between subject and object, self and world. It was in his major work *The Phenomenology of Perception* (1945) that he argued that the body had been neglected in philosophy. Because of the mind-body split in dualistic

10    Carel, *Illness*, 8.
11    Ibid.
12    M. Merleau-Ponty, *The World of Perception*, Routledge Classics (London; Routledge, 2008), 25.

thinking, the mind had been considered as separate from the body in such a way that the mind orders the body to perform tasks. Merleau-Ponty went as far as to claim that we are our bodies; there is no detachment of subject from object, or mind from body. He viewed the body and perception as the seat of personhood and subjectivity in responding to the environment. The body was no mere instrument of the mind, he said 'it is our expression in the world, the visible form of our intentions.'[13]

His theory on the unity and indivisibility of mind and body is valuable for investigating the experience of illness and, in the case of this research, the experiences of shame and stigma associated with invisible illnesses. He asserted that perception is intrinsically linked to the body. At root, a human being is a perceiving and experiencing organism, intimately inhabiting and immediately responding to her environment.[14]

In his critique of Merleau-Ponty's account of the body, David Morris has proposed that illness reveals itself not simply as an absence of the proper function of an objective body, but as a vividly experienced change in one's access to the world. This is especially the case, he has argued, in drastic chronic illness in which, 'illness changes what one can hope for, project and do in one's world, and correlatively changes the sense of oneself, even one's consciousness.'[15]

The qualitative exploratory approach utilised in this study has also been influenced by the work of Rosemarie Anderson, professor emerita of transpersonal psychology at Sofia University in California. Anderson has fostered the development of new post-positivist research methods which can do justice to the exploration of spiritual awakening in women with chronic invisible illnesses. In the early 1990s, there was a recognition in the field of spirituality research that new research methods were required that would be able to capture and describe phenomena related to spiritual experiences, altered states of consciousness and body phenomena. It was felt that 'the definition of *empirical* must eventually be expanded to

---

13   Carel, *Illness*, 25.
14   Ibid., 20.
15   D. Morris, 'Body', in *Merleau-Ponty: Key Concepts*, eds R. Diprose and J. Reynolds (Stocksfield: Acumen, 2008), 111–20.

include inner experiences, which are private and therefore unobservable by an external observer'.[16]

Anderson and her associates were critical of social scientists who copied the objectivist and positivist views of physical science: 'By owning radical positivism and psychological behaviourism as the epistemological imprimatur, psychologists and other human scientists have ignored and even trivialized vast realms of fascinating human experiences'.[17] In response to these insights, and in order to assist her doctoral students who were researching matters related to deep emotions and topics of a transpersonal nature, Rosemarie Anderson developed the research method of *intuitive inquiry*. She described intuitive inquiry as 'an interpretive research method intended for the study of subtle, and sometimes complex, human experiences'.[18] As the title suggests, intuition is at the core of the method; intuition defined as 'a facility of knowing gained through imaginable and symbolic processes, refined attention to bodily sensations, or alternative states of consciousness in contrast to rational processes.'[19] Intuition, Anderson asserted, has long been considered essential to wisdom in indigenous and spiritual traditions.

Anderson aligned with the contemplative and Harvard scholar of religion, Henri Nouwen (1932–1996), who understood human wounds to be 'sites both of suffering and hospitality to the divine'.[20] Such wounds can be transformed to become sources of inspiration for others. Intuitive inquiry may fruitfully lend itself to giving a voice to people who undergo profound shifts in consciousness due to illness. In gathering such wisdom, society as a whole can grow in wisdom from listening to those voices. In the case of this study, alertness to intuition was facilitated in the writing

---

16    R. Anderson and W. Braud, *Transforming Self and Others through Research: Transpersonal Research Methods and Skills for the Human Sciences and Humanities* (New York: SUNY Press, 2011), 3.

17    Ibid.

18    Anderson, 'Intuitive Inquiry: An Epistemology of the Heart for Scientific Inquiry', 307.

19    R. Anderson, 'Intuitive Inquiry: The Ways of the Heart in Research and Scholarship', 2006, <http://www.wellknowingconsulting.org/publications/pdfs/intuitive_inquiry_final.pdf>. Accessed 9 October 2015.

20    Anderson and Braud, *Transforming Self and Others through Research*, 25.

and analysis of a personal memoir of illness and awakening, as well as by the use of select spiritual practices.

Roberto Assagioli believed that mental and physical disturbance can be caused by energies from the Self, or the *superconscious*, influencing the personality – our higher potential calling us forth. The superconscious is the source of higher functions. It is the source of our drive for finding meaning, our values, our creative impulse, new discoveries and spiritual experiences such as those experienced by the mystics. *Process oriented psychology*, founded by Jungian analyst and psychotherapist Arnold Mindell, gives phenomenological techniques for working with this concept. Process work enabled the researcher to work with symptoms including *brain fog*, a type of cognitive dysfunction which is associated with ME/CFS. Weekly sessions in process work were undertaken for the first two years of the research. The exercises provided a lens with which illness could be viewed from a psycho-spiritual perspective. In addition, this work supported the researcher in being able to listen attentively to participants when they narrated their stories of symptoms and spiritual awakening.

Full ethical approval was gained for this research which has conformed to the highest possible standards of integrity and ethics for such research. The study adhered to ethical principles governing social inquiry including: obtaining informed consent, non-deception, absence of psychological or physical harm, respect for the privacy and confidentiality of the participants.[21] In particular this project has been guided by the ethical imperatives of non-maleficence to vulnerable groups. This is relevant to women with invisible illnesses who sometimes have their physical illness diagnosed as a mental illness when medical tests show no physical disease. This leads to hurt, stigma and trauma. The researcher was concerned that the findings of this research on the spirituality, childhood issues, or trauma of the participants could be taken out of context, thus reinforcing negative stereotypes of the group.

---

21   N. Denzin and Y. Lincoln, *Handbook of Qualitative Research*, 2nd edn (Thousand Oaks, CA: Sage Publications, 2000), 33.

# Bibliography

Alonzo, A. 'The Experience of Chronic Illness and Post-Traumatic Stress Disorder: The Consequences of Cumulative Adversity'. *Social Science & Medicine* 50, no. 10 (2000): 1475–1484.

Alsaker, S. *Narrative in Action: Meaning-Making in Everyday Activities of Women Living with Chronic Rheumatic Conditions.* Norges teknisk-naturvitenskapelige universitet, Fakultet for samfunnsvitenskap og teknologiledelse, Institutt for sosialt arbeid og helsevitenskap, 2009. <http://brage.bibsys.no/xmlui/handle/11250/267660>.

Anderson, R. 'Intuitive Inquiry: An Epistemology of the Heart for Scientific Inquiry'. *The Humanistic Psychologist* 32, no. 4 (2004): 307–41.

——. 'Intuitive Inquiry: The Ways of the Heart in Research and Scholarship', 2006. <http://www.wellknowingconsulting.org/publications/pdfs/intuitive_inquiry_final.pdf>. Accessed 9 October 2015.

Anderson, R., and W. Braud. *Transforming Self and Others through Research: Transpersonal Research Methods and Skills for the Human Sciences and Humanities.* New York: SUNY Press, 2011.

Arroll, M., and C. Dancey. *Invisible Illness: Coping with Misunderstood Conditions.* London: Sheldon Press, 2014.

Asbring, Pia, and Anna-Liisa Närvänen. 'Women's Experiences of Stigma in Relation to Chronic Fatigue Syndrome and Fibromyalgia'. *Qualitative Health Research* 12, no. 2 (February 2002): 148–60. <https://doi.org/10.1177/104973230201200202>.

Assagioli, R. *Psychosynthesis: A Collection of Basic Writings.* New York: Penguin Books, 1987.

——. *Psychosynthesis: A Manual of Principles and Techniques.* London: Viking Press, 1971.

——. 'Psychosynthesis Medicine and Bio-Psychosynthesis'. *Psychosynthesis Research Foundation*, no. 21 (1967). <http://www.psykosyntese.dk/a-147/>.

——. *Transpersonal Development.* Revised edn. Forres: Smiling Wisdom, imprint of Inner Way Productions, 2008.

Bailey Gilbert, E. *Eat, Pray, Love: One Woman's Search for Everything Across Italy, India and Indonesia.* Princeton, NJ: Penguin Books, 2007.

Beck, A. 'The Flexner Report and the Standardization of American Medical Education'. *JAMA: The Journal of the American Medical Association* 291, no. 17 (5 May 2004): 2139–40. <https://doi.org/10.1001/jama.291.17.2139>.

Ben-Zvi, A., S. Vernon, and G. Broderick. 'Model-Based Therapeutic Correction of Hypothalamic-Pituitary-Adrenal Axis Dysfunction'. *PLoS Comput Biol* 5, no. 1 (23 January 2009): 1–10. <https://doi.org/10.1371/journal.pcbi.1000273>.

Bleakley, A. 'Gender Matters in Medical Education'. *Medical Education* 47, no. 1 (January 2013): 59–70. <https://doi.org/10.1111/j.1365-2923.2012.04351.x>.

Buber, Martin. *I and Thou*. New York: Scribner, 1970.

Campbell, J. *The Hero with a Thousand Faces*. Bollingen Series ; 17. New York: Pantheon Books, 1949.

Carel, H. *Illness: The Cry of the Flesh*. Art of Living Series (Acumen Publishing). Stocksfield: Acumen, 2008.

Carel, H., and I. Kidd. 'Epistemic Injustice in Healthcare: A Philosophical Analysis'. *Medicine, Health Care, and Philosophy* 17, no. 4 (November 2014): 529–40. <https://doi.org/10.1007/s11019-014-9560-2>.

Chang, H. *Collaborative Autoethnography*. Developing Qualitative Inquiry. Walnut Creek, CA: Left Coast Press, 2012.

Charon, R. 'LitSite Alaska | Perspectives', 2000. <http://www.litsite.org/index.cfm?section=Narrative-and-Healing&page=Perspectives&viewpost=2&ContentId=985>. Accessed 26 May 2011.

——. *Narrative Medicine: Honoring the Stories of Illness*. Oxford; New York: Oxford University Press, 2006.

——. 'Preface'. In *Gender Scripts in Medicine and Narrative*, eds M. Block and A. Laflen, xiv–xviii. Newcastle upon Tyne, 2010. <http://www.cambridgescholars.com/gender-scripts-in-medicine-and-narrative-16>. Accessed 4 August 2015.

——. 'The Self-Telling Body'. *Narrative Inquiry* 16, no. 1 (2006): 191–200.

Charon, R., et al. 'Literature and Ethical Medicine: Five Cases from Common Practice'. *The Journal of Medicine and Philosophy* 21 (1996): 243–65.

Charon, R., and M. Montello. *Stories Matter: The Role of Narrative in Medical Ethics*. 1st edn. New York: Routledge, 2002.

Chernow, J. 'The Blessing of a Curse: An Examination of Growth and Transformation from Chronic Fatigue Syndrome'. Institute of Transpersonal Psychology, 2008. <http://gradworks.umi.com/33/07/3307970.html>.

Cook, C. 'Addiction and Spirituality'. *Addiction* 99, no. 5 (May 2004): 593–551.

——. 'How Spirituality Is Relevant to Mental Healthcare and Ethical Concerns', 2013. <http://www.rcpsych.ac.uk>. Accessed 7 October 2014.

Denzin, N., and Y. Lincoln. *Handbook of Qualitative Research*. 2nd edn. Thousand Oaks, CA: Sage Publications, 2000.

Donne, J. *The Works of John Donne.* J. W. Parker, 1839.

Duff, K. *The Alchemy of Illness.* New York: Harmony, 2000.

Durà-Vilà, G., S. Dein, R. Littlewood, and G. Leavey. 'The Dark Night of the Soul: Causes and Resolution of Emotional Distress among Contemplative Nuns'. *Transcultural Psychiatry* 47, no. 4 (1 September 2010): 548–70. <https://doi.org/10.1177/1363461510374899>.

Eliade, M. *Rites and Symbols of Initiation.* 1st edn. Dallas, TX; New York: Spring, 1998.

Ellenberger, H. *The Discovery of the Unconscious: The History and Evolution of Dynamic Psychiatry.* New York: Basic Books, 1970.

Engelhardt, H. 'The Birth of the Medical Humanities and the Rebirth of the Philosophy of Medicine: The Vision of Edmund D. Pellegrino'. *Journal of Medicine and Philosophy* 15, no. 3 (1 June 1990): 237–41. <https://doi.org/10.1093/jmp/15.3.237>.

Etherington, K. 'A View of Narrative Inquiry', 2003. <http://www.cprjournal.com/documents/narrativeInquiry.ppt>.

Ferrucci, P. *What We May Be: The Vision and Techniques of Psychosynthesis.* London: Aquarian Press, 1990.

Fitzgerald, C. 'Impasse and Dark Night'. In *Women's Spirituality: Resources for Christian Development*, ed. J. Wolski Conn, 287–311. New York: Paulist Press, 1988.

Flanagan, B. *Embracing Solitude: Women and New Monasticism.* Eugene, OR: Resource Publications, 2013.

Flexner, A. 'Medical Education in the United States and Canada'. New York: The Carnegie Foundation, 1910. <http://archive.carnegiefoundation.org/pdfs/elibrary/Carnegie_Flexner_Report.pdf>.

Flick, U., E. Von Kardorff, and I. Steinke. *A Companion to Qualitative Research.* Thousand Oaks, CA: Sage, 2004.

Foucault, M. *Naissance de la Clinique.* PUF edn. Paris: Presses Universitaires de France, 2000.

———. *The Order of Things: An Archaeology of the Human Sciences.* 1st edn. New York: Vintage, 1994.

Frank, A. *At the Will of the Body: Reflections on Illness.* 1st Mariner Books edn. Boston, MA: Houghton Mifflin, 2002.

———. *The Wounded Storyteller: Body, Illness, and Ethics.* Pbk edn. Chicago: University of Chicago Press, 1997.

Frankl, V. *The Will to Meaning: Foundations and Applications of Logotherapy.* Rei Exp edn. New York: Plume, 1988.

Fricker, M. *Epistemic Injustice: Power and the Ethics of Knowing.* Oxford; New York: Oxford University Press, 2007.

Fuller, R. 'Holistic Health Practices'. In *Spirituality and the Secular Quest*, ed. P van Ness, 227–50. New York: The Crossroad Publishing Company, 1996.

——. 'Subtle Energies and the American Metaphysical Tradition'. In *Religion and Healing in America*. Oxford: Oxford University Press, 2005.

Gilligan, C. *In a Different Voice: Psychological Theory and Women's Development*. Cambridge, MA; London: Harvard University Press, 1982.

Goffman, E. *Stigma: Notes on the Management of Spoiled Identity*. New York: Touchstone, 1986.

Grant, R. *The Way of the Wound: A Spirituality of Trauma and Transformation*. Burlingame, CA: self-published, 1999.

Harding, S., ed. *The Feminist Standpoint Theory Reader: Intellectual and Political Controversies*. 1st edn. New York: Routledge, 2003.

Harris, M. *Dance of the Spirit: The Seven Stages of Women's Spirituality*. Reprint edn. New York: Bantam, 1991.

Heelas, P., L. Woodhead, B. Seel, B. Szerszynski, and K. Tusting. *The Spiritual Revolution: Why Religion Is Giving Way to Spirituality*. 1st edn. Chichester: Wiley-Blackwell, 2004.

Herman, J. *Trauma and Recovery*. New York: Basic Books, 1992.

Holloway, M. 'When Medicine Meets Literature', *Scientific American*, April 2005. <http://www.scientificamerican.com/article.cfm?id=when-medicine-meets-liter&page=2>.

Johna, S., and S. Rahman. 'Humanity before Science: Narrative Medicine, Clinical Practice, and Medical Education'. *The Permanente Journal* 15, no. 4 (2011): 92–4.

Jonsen, A. *The Birth of Bioethics*. New York: Oxford University Press, 2003.

Kabat-Zinn, J. *Mindfulness for Beginners: Reclaiming the Present Moment – and Your Life*. 1st edn. Boulder, CO: Sounds True, 2011.

Kardiner, A. *The Traumatic Neuroses of War*. Atlanta, GA: National Academies, 1941.

Kavanaugh, K. *The Interior Castle Study Edition*. Reprint edn. Washington, DC: ICS Publications, 2010.

Kavanaugh, K., and E. Larkin, eds. *John of the Cross: Selected Writings*. New edn. New York: Paulist Press, 1988.

Kavanaugh, K., and O. Rodriguez. *Teresa of Avila: The Book of Her Life*. Indianapolis, IN: Hackett, 2008.

Kierkegaard, Søren. *Either/Or: A Fragment of Life*. Trans. L. Swenson and D. Swenson. Princeton, NJ: Princeton University Press, 1949.

Kleinman, A. *The Illness Narratives: Suffering, Healing, And The Human Condition*. New York: Basic Books, 1989.

——. *Patients and Healers in the Context of Culture: An Exploration of the Border-land between Anthropology, Medicine, and Psychiatry.* Berkeley: University of California Press, 1980.

——. *Rethinking Psychiatry: From Cultural Category to Personal Experience.* 1st edn. New York: Free Press, 1991.

——. 'Review: Social Origins of Distress and Disease: Depression, Neurasthenia and Pain in Modern China'. *Current Anthropology*, 5, 27, no. 5 (1 December 1986): 499–509.

Kleinman, A., and B. Good. *Culture and Depression: Studies in the Anthropology and Cross-Cultural Psychiatry of Affect and Disorder.* Oakland: University of California Press, 1986.

Koenig, H. *Handbook of Religion and Health.* Oxford; New York: Oxford University Press, 2012.

Kristeva, J. *Hatred and Forgiveness.* European Perspectives. New York: Columbia University Press, 2010.

Lancaster, L., and E. Linders. 'Sacred Illness: Exploring Transpersonal Aspects in Physi-cal Affliction and the Role of the Body in Spiritual Development'. *Mental Health* 16, no. 10 (2013): 991–1008. <https://doi.org/10.1080/13674676.2012.728578>.

Lanzetta, B. *Radical Wisdom: A Feminist Mystical Theology.* Minneapolis, MN: For-tress Press, 2005.

——. 'Women, Soul Wounds, and Integrative Medicine'. In *Integrative Women's Health*, eds V. Maizes and T. Low Dog, 84–97. Oxford: Oxford University Press, 2010.

Lynch, G. *The New Spirituality: An Introduction to Progressive Belief in the Twenty-First Century.* London; New York: I. B. Tauris, 2007.

McGinn, B. *Meister Eckhart and the Beguine Mystics: Hadewijch of Brabant, Mechthild of Magdeburg, and Marguerite Porete.* New York: The Continuum Publishing Company, 2001.

Manning, L. 'Spirituality as a Lived Experience: Exploring the Essence of Spirituality for Women in Late Life'. *International Journal of Aging & Human Development* 75, no. 2 (2012): 95–113.

Markel, H. 'Abraham Flexner and His Remarkable Report on Medical Education: A Century Later'. *JAMA: The Journal of the American Medical Association* 303, no. 9 (2 March 2010): 888–90. <https://doi.org/10.1001/jama.2010.225>.

Maslow, A. *The Farther Reaches of Human Nature.* New York: Viking Press, 1971.

——. 'A Theory of Human Motivation'. *Psychological Review* 50, no. 4 (1943): 370–96. <https://doi.org/10.1037/h0054346>.

May, G. *The Awakened Heart.* Reprint edn. San Francisco, CA: HarperOne, 1993.

——. *Care of Mind/Care of Spirit: A Psychiatrist Explores Spiritual Direction.* Reprint edn. San Francisco: HarperOne, 1992.

——. *Will and Spirit: A Contemplative Psychology*. Reprint edn. San Francisco; London: HarperOne, 1987.

Merleau-Ponty, M. *The World of Perception*. Routledge Classics. London ; Routledge, 2008.

Mindell, A. *Dreambody: The Body's Role in Revealing the Self*. 2nd edn. Portland, OR: Lao Tse Press, 1998.

——. *Metaskills: The Spiritual Art of Therapy*. Portland, OR: Lao Tse Press, 2003.

——. *The Quantum Mind and Healing: How to Listen and Respond to Your Body's Symptoms*. Charlottesville, VA: Hampton Roads Pub. Co., 2004.

——. *The Shaman's Body: A New Shamanism for Transforming Health, Relationships, and Community*. San Francisco, CA: HarperSanFrancisco, 1993.

Mishler, E. *The Discourse of Medicine: Dialectics of Medical Interviews*. New York: Ablex Publishing, 1985.

Morris, D. 'Body'. In *Merleau-Ponty: Key Concepts*, eds R. Diprose and J. Reynolds, 111–20. Stocksfield: Acumen, 2008.

Murdock, M. *The Heroine's Journey*. Boston, MA: New York: Shambhala, 1990.

Murk-Jansen, S. *Brides in the Desert: The Spirituality of the Beguines*. Traditions of Christian Spirituality. Maryknoll, NY: Orbis Books, 1998.

Newton, Benjamin J., Jane L. Southall, Jon H. Raphael, Robert L. Ashford, and Karen LeMarchand. 'A Narrative Review of the Impact of Disbelief in Chronic Pain'. *Pain Management Nursing* 14, no. 3 (September 2013): 161–71. <https://doi.org/10.1016/j.pmn.2010.09.001>.

Ogden, P. *Trauma and the Body: A Sensorimotor Approach to Psychotherapy*. 1st edn. New York: W. W. Norton & Company, 2006.

Perera, S. *Descent to the Goddess: A Way of Initiation for Women*. 1st edn. Toronto: Inner City Books, 1981.

Perkins Gilman, C. *Our Androcentric Culture*. New York: Charlton Co., 1911.

Prigogine, I., and I. Stengers. *Order out of Chaos: Man's New Dialogue with Nature*. Toronto: Bantam Books, 1984.

Pritchett, H., and A. Flexner. *Medical Education in the United States and Canada: A Report to the Carnegie Foundation for the Advancement of Teaching*. Bulletin (Carnegie Foundation for the Advancement of Teaching); No. 4. New York City: [Carnegie Foundation for the Advancement of Teaching], 1910. <http://nrs.harvard.edu/urn-3:HMS.COUNT:1181036>.

Psychosynthesis Online. 'Psychosynthesis – Free Clip Art'. Accessed 3 February 2015. <http://www.psychosynthesisonline.com/psychosynthesis-clip-art.html>.

PubMed Health. 'Patent Ductus Arteriosus'. *PubMed Health*, 11 June 2014. <https://www.ncbi.nlm.nih.gov/pubmedhealth/PMH0062968/>.

Puustinen, R., M. Leiman, and A. Viljanen. 'Medicine and the Humanities – Theoretical and Methodological Issues'. *Medical Humanities* 29, no. 2 (1 December 2003): 77–80. <https://doi.org/10.1136/mh.29.2.77>.

Robinson, A. *God and the World of Signs: Trinity, Evolution, and the Metaphysical Semiotics of C. S. Peirce.* Leiden; Boston, MA: Brill, 2010.

Romanyshyn, R. *The Wounded Researcher: Research with Soul in Mind.* New Orleans, LA: Spring Journal, Inc., 2007.

Root, M. 'Reconstructing the Impact of Trauma on Personality'. In *Personality and Psychopathology: Feminist Reappraisals*, eds L. Brown and Mary Ballou Ballou, reprint edn, 229–66. New York: The Guilford Press, 1994.

Rossman, J. *The Psychology of the Inventor: A Study of the Patentee.* New and rev. Washington, DC: Inventors Publishing, 1931.

Rudnytsky, P., and R. Charon. *Psychoanalysis and Narrative Medicine.* New York: SUNY Press, 2008.

Sandblom, P. *Creativity and Disease: How Illness Affects Literature, Art, and Music.* Rev. 7th/1st paperback. New York: Marion Boyars, 1992.

Schäfer, M. L. 'On the history of the concept neurasthenia and its modern variants chronic-fatigue-syndrome, fibromyalgia and multiple chemical sensitivities'. *Fortschritte Der Neurologie-Psychiatrie* 70, no. 11 (November 2002): 570–82. <https://doi.org/10.1055/s-2002-35174>.

Selak, J. *You Don't Look Sick!: Living Well with Invisible Chronic Illness.* New York: Haworth Medical Press, 2005.

Shapiro, J. 'Walking a Mile in Their Patients' Shoes: Empathy and Othering in Medical Students' Education'. *Philosophy, Ethics, and Humanities in Medicine*, 12 March 2008. <http://www.ncbi.nlm.nih.gov/pmc/articles/PMC2278157/>. Accessed 22 November 2012.

Simons, W. *Cities of Ladies: Beguine Communities in the Medieval Low Countries, 1200–1565.* Middle Ages Series. Philadelphia: University of Pennsylvania Press, 2001.

Slee, N. *Women's Faith Development: Patterns and Processes.* Explorations in Practical, Pastoral, and Empirical Theology. Aldershot: Ashgate, 2004.

Sontag, S. *Illness as Metaphor.* New York: Vintage Books, 1979.

Spicker, S., and R. Ratzan. 'Ars Medicina Et Conditio Humana Edmund D. Pellegrino, M. D., on His 70th Birthday'. *Journal of Medicine and Philosophy* 15, no. 3 (1 June 1990): 327–41. <https://doi.org/10.1093/jmp/15.3.327>.

Stoltzfus, M., R. Green, and D. Schumm, eds. *Chronic Illness, Spirituality, and Healing: Diverse Disciplinary, Religious, and Cultural Perspectives.* 1st edn. New York, NY: Palgrave Macmillan, 2013.

Swoboda, D. 'Embodiment and the Search for Illness Legitimacy Among Women with Contested Illnesses'. *Michigan Feminist Studies* 19 (Fall 2005): 73–90.

Thích Nhất Hạnh. *For a Future to Be Possible: Buddhist Ethics for Everyday Life.* Revised edition. Berkeley, CA: Parallax Press, 2007.

Treviño, A. J. *Goffman's Legacy.* Lanham, MD: Rowman & Littlefield, 2003.

Tyler, P. *Teresa of Avila: Doctor of the Soul.* London: Bloomsbury Academic, 2014.

Underhill, E. *Mysticism.* Oxford: One World, 1993.

——. *Mysticism: The Nature and Development of Spiritual Consciousness.* Oxford: One World, 1993.

Vachon, M. 'The Soul's Wisdom: Stories of Living and Dying'. *Current Oncology* 15, no. 0 (2008): 48–52. <https://doi.org/10.3747/co.v15i0.272>.

Velasquez, M. *Philosophy: A Text With Readings.* Boston, MA: Cengage Learning, 2010.

Wall, D. *Encounters with the Invisible: Unseen Illness, Controversy, and Chronic Fatigue Syndrome.* Dallas, TX: Southern Methodist University Press, 2005.

Ware, N. C., and A. Kleinman. 'Culture and Somatic Experience: The Social Course of Illness in Neurasthenia and Chronic Fatigue Syndrome'. *Psychosomatic Medicine* 54, no. 5 (October 1992): 546–60.

Webster's Dictionary. 'Webster's Revised Unabridged Dictionary (1913) – The ARTFL Project', 1913. <http://machaut.uchicago.edu/?resource=Webster%27s&word=neurasthenia&use1913=on>. Accessed 12 September 2015.

Welch, J. *Spiritual Pilgrims: Carl Jung and Teresa of Avila.* 1st edn. New York: Paulist Press, 1982.

Wendell, S. *The Rejected Body: Feminist Philosophical Reflections on Disability.* New York: Routledge, 1996.

Wilber, K. *Integral Spirituality: A Startling New Role for Religion in the Modern and Postmodern World.* Reprint edn. Boston, MA: Shambhala, 2007.

——. *No Boundary: Eastern and Western Approaches to Personal Growth.* Boston, MA: Shambhala, 2001.

Wilkinson, I., and A. Kleinman. *A Passion for Society: How We Think about Human Suffering.* California Series in Public Anthropology; 35. Oakland, CA: University of California Press, 2016. <http://nrs.harvard.edu/urn-3:hul.ebook:EBSCO_9780520962408>.

Yamada, K., and R. Habito. *The Gateless Gate: The Classic Book of Zen Koans.* Boston, MA: Wisdom Publications, 2004.

Zausner, T. *When Walls Become Doorways: Creativity and the Transforming Illness.* 1st edn. New York: Harmony Books, 2006.

Zimmermann, E. 'A Narrative Inquiry of Women Practitioners of Eastern Spirituality in Recovery from Childhood Trauma'. California Institute of Integral Studies, 2011. <http://gradworks.umi.com/34/90/3490158.html>.

# Index